THERAPEUTIC DRUG MONITORING AND LABORATORY MEDICINE

Mike Hallworth MA, MSc, MCB FRCPath
Consultant Clinical Scientist, Royal Shrewsbury Hospital NHS Trust,

Ian D Watson PhD, FRCPath
Consultant Clinical Scientist, Clinical Laboratories, Aintree Hospitals NHS Trust, Liverpool

Editors:
Karen Poyser MSc, PhD, FRCPath
Principal Clinical Scientist, Bronglais General Hospital, Aberystwyth

Roy Sherwood BSc, MSc, DPhil
Consultant Clinical Scientist, King's College Hospital, London

ACB VENTURE PUBLICATIONS
with generous support from Microgenics GmbH
and Siemens Medical Solutions Diagnostics

ACB VENTURE PUBLICATIONS
Chairman - Ruth Lapworth

British Library Cataloguing in Publication Data

A catalogue record for the book is available from the British Library

ISBN 978-0-902429-42-0, EAN 9780902429420, ACB Venture Publications

Printed by Piggott Black Bear (Cambridge) Ltd

Cover and illustrations by Alan Sherwood, Aspire Design Studios, London

Preface

Monitoring drug therapy has changed markedly in the 15 years since the first edition of this book. Many new drugs are now monitored, particularly in immunosuppressant therapy and the treatment of epilepsy. Established drugs such as aminoglycoside antibiotics are now used very differently than they were in 1993, and an entirely new science - pharmacogenomics - has grown up since the book was first published, and is already beginning to transform the way drugs are used. Some of the drugs deemed worthy of monitoring in the last century are now rarely encountered, having been replaced with more effective drugs which do not require the same degree of surveillance. We hope this new edition reflects these changes and will continue to prove useful to clinicians, pharmacists and laboratory scientists.

There have been a number of changes to the team behind the book for this edition. Nigel Capps has moved on, and Ian Watson joins Mike Hallworth as a principal author. We are extremely grateful to Professor David Holt and Professor Atholl Johnston (London) who have jointly contributed the sections on immunosuppressants and cardioactive drugs. Dr Steve Soldin (Washington DC) also made valuable comments on the first edition text.

We also thank our editors, Karen Poyser and Roy Sherwood, whose skill is exceeded only by their patience, and Alan Sherwood for the illustrations. We are deeply grateful for the unfailing support of our wives, Barbara and Alison, throughout the writing process.

Mike Hallworth
Ian Watson
April 2008

Acknowledgements

The authors are grateful to the following for permission to reproduce or adapt material for certain figures used in this publication:

American Medical Association, Dubois *et al* Arch Int Med 1916; **17:** 863-871 (Appendix Figs 1 & 2)

American Society for Microbiology, Nicolau *et al*, Antimicrob Agents Chemo 1995; **29:** 650-655 (Figure 4.8).

Elsevier, Koch-Weser J, 1981; 1-22 in Therapeutic Drug Monitoring. Eds. Richens A, Marks V (Figure 1.1)

Elsevier, Mullen PW, Clin Pharmacol Ther 1978; **23:** 229-232 (Figure 4.6)

Elsevier, Rambeck B, Ther Drug Monit 1979; **1:** 325-333 (Figure 4.5)

Elsevier, Siersbaek-Nielsen K *et al*, Lancet 1971; **1:** 1133-1134 (Appendix Figure 3)

John Wiley & sons, Jusko WJ *et al* J Pharmaceutic Sci 1979; **68:** 1358-1366. Copyright (1979) American Pharmacists Association, reprinted with permission of Wiley-Liss inc a subsidiary of John Wiley & sons inc. (Figure 4.3)

Royal Society of Medicine Press, Chrystyn H *et al* 1984; **78:** 117-126 in New Perspectives in Theophylline Therapy, Eds. Turner-Warwick M & Levy J (Figure 4.4)

Springer-Verlag, Vozeh S *et al*, J Pharmacokinet (Biopharm) Pharmacodynam 1981; **9:** 131-146 (Figure 4.7)

Contents

Chapter 1

Theoretical considerations

Introduction

Therapeutic drug monitoring (TDM) is the use of drug measurements in body fluids as an aid to the management of drug therapy for the cure, alleviation or prevention of disease. It has long been customary to adjust the dosage of drugs according to the characteristics of the individual being treated and the response obtained, and physicians have been most ready to do this when the pharmacological response can be easily established by clinical means (e.g. antihypertensive drugs, analgesics, hypnotics), or by laboratory markers (e.g. anticoagulants, hypoglycaemic agents, lipid-lowering drugs, hormone preparations). If there is a wide margin between the toxic dose and the therapeutically effective dose, then monitoring may be unnecessary (e.g. penicillins). However, where this is not the case and the drug's action cannot readily be assessed clinically (e.g. in the prophylaxis of seizures or mania), or when toxic effects cannot be detected until severe or irreversible (e.g. aminoglycoside antibiotics, immunosuppressants), then dosage individualisation is much more difficult, though no less important. TDM now has an established place in enabling optimisation of therapy with such agents, although it must be emphasised that clinical and other criteria remain important and TDM should never be the sole basis for individualisation of therapy. TDM has been established for a tightly defined group of drugs and must be considered as a process that begins with a clinical question and continues by devising a sampling strategy to answer that question, measuring one or more drug concentrations using a suitable method and interpreting the results appropriately.

Although TDM has been routinely practised in clinical laboratories since the mid-1970s, the scientific foundations of the subject can be traced to the late 1930s when Teorrell laid the foundations for determination of the kinetics of exogenously administered substances. This enables dose to be predicted given knowledge of distribution and clearance. In the next decade, Marshall, in studies of antibiotics, first tested the concept that the activity of a drug was dependent on its concentration. Buchthal showed in 1960 that there was a relationship between plasma concentrations of phenytoin in patients being treated for epilepsy and the degree of seizure control attained, and Baastrup and Schou demonstrated the relationship between plasma concentration and pharmacological effect for lithium in 1967. This work coincided with the rise of clinical pharmacology as an independent discipline during the 1960s, and the development of the fundamental concepts of pharmacokinetics and pharmacodynamics.

The scene was thus set for the surge of publications in the early 1970s on improving individualisation of therapy by monitoring of drug concentrations and appropriate adjustment of dose – the beginnings of TDM as we know it. The remaining barrier to widespread adoption of the concept, the availability of appropriate analytical methods, was removed in the mid-1970s by the commercial application of the homogeneous enzyme immunoassay technique developed by Rubinstein, Schneider and Ullman and marketed by the Syva Company as EMIT. The ability to provide accurate and precise results simply and quickly and the pioneering work of Syva in educating doctors and medical scientists in the advantages of TDM as an aid to individualisation of therapy, resulted in the explosive growth of TDM applications in the second half of the 1970s. In retrospect, this growth was perhaps too rapid, outstripping an understanding of the theoretical and practical considerations necessary to ensure that the measurements were correctly applied and interpreted.

Spector divided the history of TDM into three distinct phases. Initially the principles were broadly accepted and the technique extensively applied to a large variety of drugs and clinical circumstances; then specific criteria were established which defined and limited the types of drug and clinical situations in which TDM was likely to be most effective, and finally (the present phase) critical evaluation of the costs and clinical benefit of TDM by means of well-controlled prospective clinical trials (which were unfortunately rare during the initial development of the subject). The remainder of this chapter will introduce some of the theoretical concepts necessary for an understanding of TDM and discuss some findings of the second and third phases of its development.

Why is TDM necessary?

As stated above, there are a number of drugs whose desired (or toxic) effects cannot readily be assessed clinically, but are related to the amount of drug in the body. In such cases, the logical approach to control the effect of the drug is to limit the amount that is given to the patient. Pragmatically this can be done by using standard doses that will produce a satisfactory response in the majority of patients – an approach that historically has been widely used in medicine and is undoubtedly effective for a large number of drugs, e.g. penicillins. The advent of pharmacogenomics is poised to change the 'one dose fits all' paradigm, and will be discussed further in Chapter 5.

For many (but not all) drugs, the primary determinant of clinical response is the concentration that can be achieved at the site of action (the cell receptor, locus of infection, etc). Often, wide variations in drug concentration above a minimum or threshold level will make little difference to the clinical effect. However, for some drugs the desired effect (and various unwanted effects) may be very sensitive to the drug concentration at a given time. Dr Bernard Brodie suggested in a keynote lecture given in 1967 that the marked heterogeneity of biological species with regard to drug metabolism meant that it would be preferable to relate drug effects to the plasma drug concentration rather than the dose.

The problem with an approach based on standard dosing for some drugs is illustrated in Figure 1.1, which shows the frequency distribution of plasma phenytoin concentrations among 200 ambulatory patients chronically treated with 300 mg/day. If we accept 5-20 mg/L (20-80 µmol/L) as the range over which phenytoin exerts a clinically useful effect (this point will be discussed later in the book), it is clear that a large number of patients receiving the standard dose have plasma phenytoin concentrations below those said to be effective, and a minority have concentrations significantly above the generally accepted range and may be exhibiting features of toxicity.

Distribution of plasma phenytoin concentrations

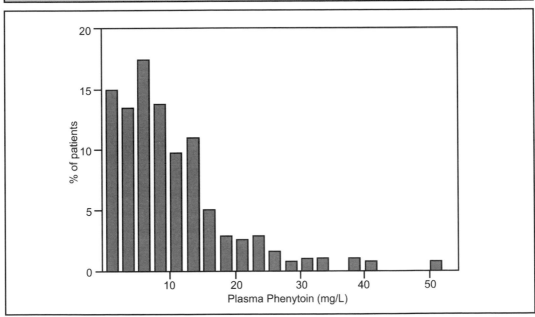

Figure 1.1 Frequency distribution of plasma phenytoin concentrations in 200 adult outpatients taking phenytoin (300 mg/day). Koch-Weser J. 'Serum drug concentrations in clinical perspective' In: Richens A, Marks V (eds). Therapeutic Drug Monitoring. Edinburgh: Churchill Livingstone 1981: 1-22 with permission.

The steady state phenytoin concentration in a given patient clearly cannot be predicted from the dose, due to inter-individual variation in the processes which are involved between prescribing a drug and that drug achieving an effective concentration at its site of action. These processes are summarised in Figure 1.2, and will now be discussed in more detail. They are conveniently divided into pharmacokinetic factors and pharmacodynamic factors. Essentially, pharmacokinetics may be defined as what the body does to drugs (the processes of absorption, distribution, metabolism and excretion) and pharmacodynamics as what the drugs do to the body (mechanisms of drug action and biochemical/physiological effects).

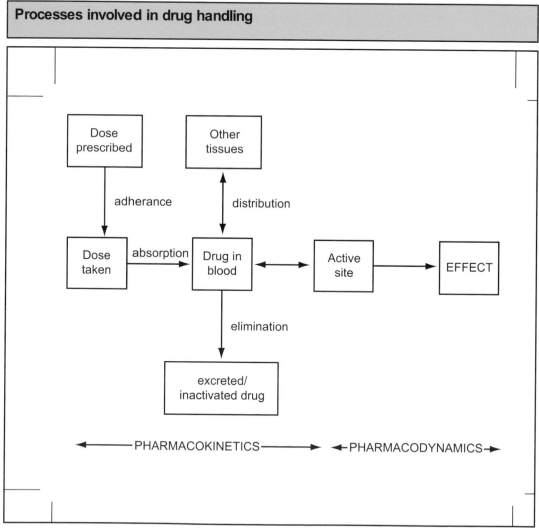

Processes involved in drug handling

Figure 1.2 Processes involved in drug handling

Adherance (Compliance)

The first potential problem affecting the relationship between prescribed dose and clinical effect is the question of whether the patient actually takes the drug as prescribed. Patients are highly motivated to comply with medication when in the acute stages of a painful or debilitating illness, but as they recover and the purpose of medication becomes prophylactic, it is easy for them to underestimate its importance and adopt a more cavalier attitude to medication. The prescribed regime may only be followed when symptoms recur or an out-patient appointment looms.

Adherence to the prescribed regime has traditionally been termed *compliance*, but in recent years the term *adherance* has been considered to be less perjorative and more consistent with the idea of partnership between the patient and clinician. This concept is particularly important in chronic disease states such as asthma, epilepsy, diabetes or manic-depressive psychosis, where variable *adherance* with the prescribed regime is widespread.

The fact that a patient is not taking a prescribed drug at all is readily detectable by measurement of drug concentration, although variable *adherance* may be more difficult to prove. Whether the assessment of *adherance* is justification in itself for TDM assays remains controversial, and will be discussed later in this chapter.

Pharmacokinetic factors

Bioavailability

Once a drug has actually been taken orally, the next potential source of variation relates to the amount of the dose that reaches the circulation. Drugs given orally may exhibit considerable variation in the percentage that is absorbed, and this factor is termed the bioavailability (F) of a drug. Bioavailability is simply defined as the fraction of dose that reaches the systemic circulation:

$$F \quad = \quad \frac{\text{dose reaching circulation}}{\text{dose administered}} \qquad\qquad \text{Eq. 1.1}$$

Bioavailability varies not only between drugs, but also between individuals and between different dosage forms of the same drug (in the case of intravenous dosing, all the administered drug is delivered to the circulation and bioavailability = 100% by definition). The two aspects of bioavailability are the formulation of the drug (e.g. the type of salt or the excipient [packing material] that has been used) and the intra- and inter-individual variation in absorption of equal doses. In the former case, there are many examples where an apparently small change to the formulation of a drug has led to large changes in bioavailability and consequently major effects on the plasma concentration and clinical effect. In Australia, in 1968, a large number of cases of phenytoin toxicity were reported in patients who had previously been well controlled. The cause was eventually traced to a change in the excipient used in a particular brand of tablets, which had markedly increased the bioavailability of the drug. Similar problems have been reported for digoxin formulations in the past. Alternatively, co-administration of foods or other drugs (especially antacids, antidiarrhoeal agents and chelating agents) and the integrity and function of the gastrointestinal tract (motility, gastric and intestinal pH) or genetic variability in absorption may affect bioavailability. When the drug is given as tablets or capsules, bioavailability may be affected by their dissolution properties in the gut.

It is important to stress that bioavailability is a measure of the *extent* to which a drug is absorbed, and gives no information about the *rate* of absorption. A drug may be slowly but completely absorbed and hence still have high bioavailability. Rate of absorption is only relevant to bioavailability if it is so slow that the drug passes through the gut before absorption is complete. This is sometimes the case with sustained release preparations.

Other routes of administration such as intramuscular, subcutaneous or sub-lingual may also exhibit incomplete bioavailability e.g. in the case of intramuscular injection local factors may lead to sequestration of drug at the injection site so that a significant proportion never reaches the circulation.

First-pass metabolism

Even after the drug has been absorbed from the gastrointestinal tract, systemic bioavailability may be reduced by metabolic transformation in the gut wall or by first-pass metabolism. Blood from the gut passes directly to the liver before reaching other major organs. If a drug is efficiently removed in the liver a significant fraction may be lost on the first pass and never reach the desired site of action. Drugs characterised by high hepatic clearance include tricyclic antidepressants, lidocaine and opiate analgesics.

Variations in bioavailability clearly have a marked influence on plasma drug concentration, and therefore drugs that fall into this category because of variable formulations or differences in absorption (e.g. theophylline) are potentially suitable candidates for TDM.

Salt-conversion factor

Another property which, although strictly unrelated to bioavailability, is frequently considered at the same time is the molecular form of the drug that is actually being administered. For example, phenytoin may be given as the free acid (MW 252 daltons) or as the sodium salt (MW 274 daltons), and the concentration of active moiety is obviously different w/w (100 mg phenytoin is equivalent to 108 mg phenytoin sodium).

This is also the case for theophylline (frequently administered as the EDTA chelate, aminophylline; 200 mg aminophylline is equivalent to 160 mg theophylline), and lithium, which may be prescribed as the carbonate or the citrate (200 mg lithium carbonate is equivalent to 520 mg lithium citrate). Changing from a given dose of one form to an equal mass of another form may result in considerable differences in plasma concentration. The fraction of active drug present in a particular salt or compound is sometimes referred to as the *salt conversion factor* or *salt fraction*.

The quantity of active drug reaching the systemic circulation is therefore related to the mass of the dosage form by the bioavailability (F) and the salt fraction (S), i.e.:

$$\text{Dose of drug absorbed} = S \times F \times (\text{Dose administered}) \qquad \text{Eq. 1.2}$$

Distribution

Once drugs have reached the systemic circulation, the process of distribution to other compartments of the body begins. The extent of distribution of a drug is governed by its relative solubility in fat and water, and by the binding capabilities of the drug to plasma proteins and tissue lipids. Drugs which are strongly bound to plasma proteins and exhibit low lipid solubility and tissue binding will show minimal distribution into tissue fluids. Conversely, high lipid solubility and tissue binding combined with low binding to plasma proteins will result in a drug being widely distributed throughout the body. The pharmacokinetic parameter that is used to describe the distribution of a drug is the apparent volume of distribution, V_d. This is defined as the volume of a compartment necessary to account for the total amount of a drug in the body if it were present throughout the compartment at the same concentration found in the plasma at a given time.

In mathematical terms,

$$\text{Volume of distribution } (V_d) = \frac{\text{Amount of drug in body}}{\text{Concentration in plasma}} \qquad \text{Eq. 1.3}$$

For example, if we know that a body contains 1000 mg of a particular drug and the plasma concentration is 20 mg/L, the apparent volume of distribution is $1000/20 = 50$ L at the time in question. It is important to realize that volume of distribution is a theoretical concept, and has no relationship to an actual physical space. The fact that apparent volumes of distribution for highly lipophilic drugs far exceed total body volume (e.g. amiodarone, V_d = approx 5000 L in a 70 kg man) illustrates this point well.

After reaching the systemic circulation, many drugs exhibit a distribution phase during which the drug concentration in each compartment reaches equilibrium. This may be rapid (approximately 15 minutes for the aminoglycoside antibiotics) or prolonged (at least six hours for digoxin). There is generally little point in taking measurements during the distribution phase (except if poisoning is suspected), although the effective drug concentration clearly depends on whether the receptor or site of action for clinical or toxic effects is in contact with the plasma itself (e.g. lidocaine) or with tissue fluids (e.g. digoxin).

Apparent volume of distribution varies between drugs according to their physical properties and other factors (Figure 1.3) and between individuals according to physical size, amount of adipose tissue and the presence of disease (e.g. ascites). Between-patient variation in volume of distribution makes a significant contribution to the poor relationship between dose and plasma concentration described at the beginning of this section.

Factors affecting distribution of drugs
Plasma protein binding
Active transport mechanisms
Tissue binding   - lipid solubility   - number and affinity of receptor sites
Regional blood flow (for drugs with high extraction ratios)
Disease

Figure 1.3 Some factors affecting distribution of drugs

Metabolism and Excretion

When a drug has been completely distributed throughout its volume of distribution, the concentration can only be maintained if the rate of administration exactly balances the rate of loss. The two processes which govern loss of drug from the body are metabolism (usually in the liver) and excretion (usually via the kidneys into the urine or via the liver into the bile). Both processes are encompassed by the pharmacokinetic parameter known as clearance (Cl), which reflects the ability of the organs of elimination to remove drug from the body. Clearance is expressed in terms of the theoretical volume of blood that can be completely cleared of drug in unit time (cf. creatinine clearance). Since at steady state the rates of administration and elimination of drug must be equal, and since clearance is defined as the proportionality constant between elimination rate and plasma concentration, it follows that:

$$\text{Rate of administration} = Cl \times Cp_{ss} \quad \text{(rate of elimination)} \qquad \text{Eq. 1.4}$$

where Cp_{ss} = mean plasma concentration at steady state.

It should now be clear that the amount of drug removed from the body in any given period is a function of plasma concentration as well as clearance. Since the average rate of administration of a drug is simply given by the dose (corrected for bioavailability and salt fraction if necessary – see above) divided by the time between doses, Equation 1.4 can be expressed as:

$$\frac{\text{Dose} \times S \times F}{\tau} = Cl \times Cp_{ss} \qquad \text{Eq. 1.5}$$

(where τ represents the interval between doses)

Or,

$$\text{Clearance} = \frac{\text{Dose} \times S \times F}{\tau \times Cp_{ss}} \qquad \text{Eq. 1.6}$$

If an estimate of the clearance of a drug can be obtained from the literature, then Eq. 1.5 can be rearranged to yield an expression which allows prediction of a maintenance dose which will produce a desired average plasma concentration at steady state:

$$\text{Maintenance dose} = \frac{Cl \times Cp_{ss} \times \tau}{S \times F} \qquad \text{Eq. 1.7}$$

Dosage prediction is described in more detail in Chapter 4.

The factors affecting clearance are summarised in Figure 1.4 and include renal and hepatic function, and the blood supply to these organs (which depends on cardiac output). Body size also affects clearance, and may be expressed in terms of weight or surface area. Clearance measurements should be corrected for body weight or surface area when relating data obtained from different individuals. Changes in the degree of plasma protein binding of a drug will also affect the apparent clearance obtained from Eq. 1.6, if total drug concentrations in plasma are used. This effect is discussed in the next section.

Factors affecting clearance
Body weight
Body surface area
Plasma protein binding
Renal function
Hepatic function
Cardiac output
Other drugs competing with metabolising enzymes

Figure 1.4 Some factors affecting clearance

The definition of clearance, (see Eq. 1.4 on page 9) implies that the rate of elimination is directly proportional to drug concentration, provided that the proportionality constant (clearance) does not itself vary with concentration. This is effectively true for a large number of drugs, which are said to be described by first-order kinetics, i.e. a constant percentage of drug is removed per unit of time whatever the plasma concentration. The elimination of drug is described by first-order decay equations, similar to those applied to radioactive decay (also a first-order process). Defining the elimination rate constant, k_{el}, as the percentage elimination per unit time, the equation for removal of drug from the circulation is:

$$A = A_0 \times e^{-k_{el}t} \qquad \text{Eq. 1.8}$$

where A = amount of drug in the body at time t
and A_0 = amount of drug present at zero time.

Since k_{el} is defined as the percentage of the total amount of drug in the body that is cleared in unit time, it may be expressed as:

$$k_{el} \quad = \quad \frac{\text{Amount cleared in unit time}}{\text{Total amount in body}}$$

$$= \quad \frac{Cl \times Cp}{V_d \times Cp} \qquad \text{(from eqns 1.3 and 1.4)}$$

$$= \quad \frac{Cl}{V_d} \qquad\qquad\qquad \text{Eq. 1.9}$$

The elimination rate constant is often expressed in terms of the elimination half-life of a drug, which is easier to apply in clinical situations. Half life ($t_{1/2}$) is the time required for the amount of drug in the body to fall to half its original value, i.e.:

$$\frac{A}{2} \quad = \quad A \times e^{-k_{el}t_{1/2}}$$

$$\ln(1/2) \quad = \quad -k_{el} \times t_{1/2}$$

$$t_{1/2} \quad = \quad \frac{0.693}{k_{el}} \qquad\qquad \text{Eq. 1.10}$$

$$(0.693 = \ln 2)$$

When clearance mechanisms become saturated there is a disproportionate increase in plasma concentration for progressive dose increments and kinetics cease to be first-order and become zero-order. This is discussed further in Chapter 4.

Plasma protein binding
Just as many endogenous constituents of the plasma circulate bound to protein (e.g. bilirubin, cortisol, some hormones), so drugs are frequently also carried by binding proteins (usually albumin and α_1-acid glycoprotein [orosomucoid]). Examples of the variable protein binding exhibited by drugs are shown in Figure 1.5.

Protein binding of drugs	
Drug	**% protein bound in plasma**
Lithium	0
Gentamicin	<10
Digoxin	20
Theophylline	60
Carbamazepine	70-80
Phenytoin	90-94
Mycophenolic acid	98

Figure 1.5 Examples of protein binding of drugs

It is generally assumed (though with little experimental justification) that the clinical effect of a drug and the processes of metabolism and excretion are controlled only by the free form of the drug, and that the fraction bound to protein is inert. However, the binding affinity will also impact on the availability of drug to interact with receptors and the amount of drug available for excretion or metabolism, which will in turn result in differing concentrations of total drug in plasma for a given dose and a given value for clearance. The free concentrations of drug under these conditions (other factors being equal) would be identical. The free fraction of a drug is defined as follows:

$$\text{Free fraction} = \frac{\text{Unbound drug}}{\text{Total drug}}$$

Eq. 1.11

Variations in the degree of protein binding can be caused by changes in the concentration of binding proteins, especially in disease states (e.g. nephrotic syndrome, acute phase reactions), by the presence of other drugs or endogenous substances (e.g. in renal failure) that compete for the same binding sites on protein or cause a modification of protein binding sites e.g. in diabetes. For these reasons, it has been suggested that the free concentrations of drugs rather than their total concentrations, should be measured for the purposes of a TDM service, at least for those drugs exhibiting significant protein binding, e.g. phenytoin. The situation is analogous to the use of free hormone measurements in endocrinology, but despite the apparent logic of the idea, it has not been generally adopted for TDM, because of methodological difficulties and continuing controversy over whether measurements of free drug concentrations actually show better concentration/effect relationships than those of the total. It is nonetheless important to be aware of the effects of protein binding changes when interpreting total drug concentrations in plasma, especially in situations where the free fraction of a drug may change within an individual over time, e.g. in pregnancy, acute illness, with changing renal function, and when other drugs are being administered. In some cases, the free fraction of a drug in plasma varies with the concentration, which makes total concentration measurements very difficult to interpret. Sodium valproate is a good example (see page 65).

Pharmacodynamic factors

The preceding discussion has outlined the pharmacokinetic factors that influence the relationship between dose and plasma concentration, showing how these may vary between patients to make dose a poor predictor of plasma concentration. Once at steady state concentration in plasma, however, the drug still has to exert its effect at a particular site of action. As indicated earlier, the time interval between reaching steady state in plasma and at the receptor may be variable, but in general once steady state is well established the concentration at the site of action should reflect that in plasma. This may not be the case if the blood supply to tissue is impaired, e.g. for poorly vascularised tissues or a tumour that has outgrown its blood supply (cytotoxics), or a locus of infection that is not well served by blood vessels (antibiotics). Between-individual variations in receptor binding or in diffusion rates across membranes may also contribute to differences between the concentrations found in plasma and at the site of action.

Pharmacodynamics is the study of the relationship between the concentration of drug at the site of action and the nature and intensity of its effect. The responsiveness of the receptor may be affected by pathological disturbances (e.g. hypokalaemia), the presence of other drugs competing for the same receptor or the functional state of the receptor itself. Reduction in target receptor affinity is a well recognised mechanism by which bacteria acquire antibiotic resistance. Marked inter-individual variability in pharmacodynamics may be genetically determined or reflect developed tolerance; this severely limits the utility of monitoring drug concentrations in such circumstances.

Criteria for valid TDM: which drugs?

Having reviewed the pharmacokinetic factors which affect drug handling, we are now in a position to define criteria for drug concentration monitoring to be a valuable adjunct to therapy. The essential criteria are summarised in Figure 1.6.

Criteria for valid TDM
Poor correlation between dose and effect
Narrow concentration interval between toxic and therapeutic effect
Absence of good clinical markers of effect
Good correlation between plasma drug concentration and effect
- low pharmacodynamic variability
- no active metabolites or metabolites measurable
- reversible action at the receptor site

Figure 1.6 Criteria for valid TDM

Poor correlation between dose and effect

Self-evidently, if the dose is a good predictor of pharmacological effect, then dose can be used to monitor therapy and TDM is not normally required. TDM is primarily of benefit where there is poor correlation between dose and effect (wide inter-individual pharmacokinetic variation).

Narrow concentration interval between therapeutic and toxic effects

The *therapeutic index* (therapeutic ratio, toxic-therapeutic ratio) is usually defined in animal studies as the dose that produces toxicity (toxic dose, TD50) or death (lethal dose, LD50) in 50% of a group of animals, divided by the dose that produces the desired effect in 50% of subjects (effective dose, ED50). This definition is of little use in clinical studies, where a more conservative definition must be used, such as the ratio of the dose that produces serious toxicity in a very small percentage of patients (say TD1) and the dose that produces a satisfactory effect in the vast majority (say ED95). It is perhaps better to use the concept in a qualitative sense as indicating the margin between the therapeutic dose and the toxic dose; the larger, the better. For most patients (with the exception of those who are hypersensitive) penicillin has a very high therapeutic index and it is safe to use in much higher doses than necessary to treat the patient satisfactorily, with no necessity to check the concentration attained. However, for other drugs (e.g. anti-coagulants, aminoglycoside antibiotics, some anti-neoplastic drugs, immuno-suppressants, cardiac glycosides) the margin between desirable and toxic dose is very small and monitoring is valuable in achieving effective concentrations and minimising the risk of toxicity.

Absence of clinical markers of effect

TDM is clearly of little value when the desired effect and any associated adverse effects can readily be quantitated by simple clinical measurements, (e.g. blood pressure in the case of antihypertensive agents or plasma glucose concentration for oral hypoglycaemic drugs). While plasma concentration data for such drugs are valuable in their development to define a pharmacokinetic profile and dosing regimen, TDM will not be helpful in the routine management of patients, except in the elucidation of rare cases where a high dose of drug fails to produce the desired effect. In such circumstances, TDM may help in differentiating poor *adherance*, poor drug absorption, receptor dysfunction or the use of the wrong drug for the situation.

Good correlation between plasma concentration and effect

This is the fundamental condition which must be fulfilled if TDM is going to be useful for a particular drug. The concentration measurements must give accurate information about the biological effect, otherwise they are of no value and may even be misleading. Plasma concentrations should correlate well with effect or toxicity, and thereby define the therapeutic window and allow titration of the dose to achieve a given effect. Demonstration of a close concentration-effect relationship requires that there is minimal between-individual pharmacodynamic variability (see p.13), no metabolites which contribute to the biological effect but are not measured in the assay system and a reversible mode of action at the receptor site.

Active metabolites are a feature of the action of many drugs, some of which may in fact be pro-drugs i.e. the parent compound has zero or minimal activity. In such cases, pharmacological activity is exclusively resident in the product(s) of metabolic transformation e.g. mycophenolate mofetil is metabolised to the active immunosuppressive agent mycophenolate. It will be clear that useful information cannot be obtained from concentration measurements if a substantial fraction of the effects of a drug is mediated by a metabolite which is not measured and whose concentration relationship to the parent compound is undefined. For some drugs, the activity of a metabolite is well understood and quantitatively similar to that of the parent drug. In such cases, both drug and metabolite concentrations may be measured and the concentrations summed to give a combined indication of effect.

This approach is useful for some of the tricyclic antidepressants and their desmethyl derivatives (e.g. amitriptyline and nortriptyline, imipramine and desipramine). For other drugs with active metabolites, the metabolite concentrations are better determined and expressed separately, (e.g. carbamazepine 10,11 epoxide and trans-diol).

If an effective relationship between concentration and effect is to be demonstrated, the intensity and the duration of the pharmacodynamic response to a drug must be temporally correlated with the concentration at the receptor site. This is only possible if the drug exhibits a reversible interaction with its receptor i.e., the binding of drug to the receptor is reversible, and the clinical effect ceases when the drug is no longer present at the receptor.

Some drugs exert irreversible effects at their receptors. For example, reserpine acts by depleting synapses of monoamines by interfering with intracellular storage. The cytotoxic alkylating agents form chemical bonds at their site of action and cannot be removed, while the anticonvulsant vigabatrin acts as a suicide substrate for the enzyme γ-aminobutyric acid transaminase and is metabolised to a compound which irreversibly inactivates the enzyme. Such drugs may not develop their clinical effect until some time after peak concentrations have been attained, and the effect may persist for days or weeks after the drug becomes undetectable in the blood. Studies on the effect of sodium valproate on the photo-convulsive response in man have shown persistence of the suppressive effect up to five days after sodium valproate is no longer detectable in the plasma. For drugs such as these, where there is no close temporal relationship between concentration and effect, it is very difficult to use plasma concentration measurements to guide therapy. The exception to this general rule may be some anti-cancer agents, where the action of the drug is irreversible, but an index of the body's total exposure to the drug may predict subsequent response.

The list of drugs which fulfil the criteria listed in Figure 1.6 is small (see upper portion of Figure 1.7). Phenytoin and lithium are probably the best and earliest examples of drugs that meet all the criteria and for which TDM is essential. The aminoglycoside antibiotics, chiefly gentamicin and tobramycin, also qualify on all counts. Theophylline meets most criteria, although its clinical effects are slightly easier to assess, in adults at least, and its clinical use continues to decline. A number of other drugs which are frequently monitored fail to meet one or more criteria completely, and the effectiveness of TDM as an aid to management is therefore severely reduced. The concentration-effect relationship for carbamazepine is not always straightforward because of the presence of active metabolites. Digoxin fulfils most of the criteria, but with some doubt about the concentration-effect relationship.

Drugs suitable for TDM

Drugs of established value

Aminoglycoside antibiotics (amikacin, gentamicin, netilmicin, tobramycin)
Carbamazepine
Ciclosporin
Digoxin
Lamotrigine
Lithium
Methadone
Methotrexate
Mycophenolate
Phenytoin
Tacrolimus
Theophylline
Vancomycin

Less well established but useful in some circumstances

Amiodarone
Anti-retroviral drugs (azathioprine, protease inhibitors etc)
Caffeine
Chloramphenicol
Clozapine
Disopyramide
Flecainide
Flucytosine
Olanzapine
Phenobarbital
Procainamide (+ NAPA)
Quinidine
Sirolimus
Tricyclic antidepressants (amitriptyline/nortriptyline, imipramine/desipramine, dothiepin)
Valproate

Figure 1.7 Drugs suitable for TDM

In the case of sodium valproate, good evidence for a concentration-effect relationship for either its anticonvulsant or thymoleptic effects is scanty. The drug has few concentration-dependent toxic effects, and there is little point in measuring its plasma concentration except in detailed pharmacokinetic studies and for the detection of gross non-adherance, particularly in psychiatric applications, or the confirmation of self-poisoning. These points are discussed further in Chapter 2.

The evidence for many drugs is based more on practical experience than well designed studies. However, when the immunosuppressant ciclosporin was introduced into clinical practice, considerable effort was invested in demonstrating the beneficial outcomes associated with effective TDM; this has provided a model for subsequent immunosuppressants e.g. tacrolimus, sirolimus and mycophenolate. Similar evidence is accumulating to support the benefit of TDM for anti-retroviral drugs.

Essentials for effective TDM – Practical considerations

Once the narrow range of drugs for which TDM can provide useful information has been defined, it should not be assumed that TDM is therefore required for all patients receiving these drugs. For a concentration measurement to be applied effectively to improve patient care, six criteria must be satisfied on each occasion a sample is taken. These are set out in Figure 1.8.

Criteria for effective drug monitoring

Rational indication for request

Accurate patient information

Appropriate sample

Accurate analysis

Correct interpretation

Appropriate response

Figure 1.8 Criteria for effective drug monitoring

Indication for request

The first essential for making effective use of any laboratory test is to be clear from the outset what question is being asked. This is particularly true of TDM requests, and the widespread failure to define the indication for analysis is at the root of most of the problems faced by TDM services. If it is not clear what the question is, or if it is the wrong question, then the answer is of little value.

The main reasons for measuring drugs in blood may be summarised as:

(a) to ensure that sufficient drug is reaching the drug receptor to produce the desired response (which may be delayed in onset),
(b) to ensure that drug (or metabolite) concentrations are not so high as to produce symptoms or signs of toxicity,
(c) to guide dosage adjustment in clinical situations in which the pharmaco-kinetics are changing rapidly (e.g. in neonates, children or patients in whom hepatic or renal function is changing),
(d) to define the pharmacokinetic parameters and concentration-effect relation-ships of new drugs.

A fifth indication, the assessment of adherence (compliance) as an indication for TDM is still to some extent controversial. Clearly, if it were accepted as a valid indication there could be a requirement to provide a service for virtually every drug in the pharmacopoeia, at enormous cost. Further, although gross non-adherence is readily detectable by TDM, variable adherence may be difficult or impossible to detect, and the very variability in pharmacokinetics that makes TDM necessary also implies that surprisingly low plasma concentrations for a given dose of drug are not necessarily due to poor adherence with the prescribed regime. Much harm has been done to the practice of TDM and to the doctor-patient relationship by over-ready assumptions of poor adherence when concen-tration measurements show unexpectedly low blood drug concentrations. Adherence may be assessed in other ways, by tablet counting, supervised medica-tion during a spell in hospital or by the use of carefully designed questions that are non-judgmental, e.g. "How often do you forget to take your tablets?". Interventional reinforcement such as this shows the patient that the clinician 'cares' and improves efforts to adhere with the agreed regimen. Such approaches are likely to be more effective than TDM. Concentration monitoring may be considered in patients with poor symptom control who deny poor adherence despite careful questioning and reinforcement.

Appropriate patient information

The requirement for specific information about patients to enable appropriate interpretation of TDM results has in the past led many hospitals to design request forms specifically for TDM analyses. Such forms normally include direct questions relating to the fundamental information requirements for TDM (see Figure 1.9). More recently, service rationalisations have resulted in multi-purpose forms which make collecting specific information more difficult, and workload and staffing pressures often mean that policing inadequate requests is challenging if not impossible. However, with the increasing use of computerised order-entry systems, essential items of clinical information can be made mandatory at the point of requesting, and linked to rule-bases to improve use of the service.

Information requirements for TDM requests		
	Essential	**Desirable**
Patient	Name Age Sex Hospital/NHS number Pathology	Weight Renal/hepatic function
Problem	Toxicity? Poor response?	
Therapy	Drug of interest - dose - length of therapy - date/time of last dose - formulation and route of administration	Other drugs - list all
Sample	Date and time taken	

Figure 1.9 Information requirements for TDM requests

Appropriate sample

An appropriate specimen is obviously a prime necessity for effective TDM. This requires that the patient is at steady state on the present dose of the drug, except when suspected toxicity is being investigated, when waiting to attain steady state is clearly contraindicated. The time taken to reach steady state is determined by the plasma half-life of the drug, and the relationship between the number of half-lives elapsed and the progress towards steady state concentrations is shown in Figure 1.10.

Percentage of steady state at various times	
Time (half-life)	**% steady state**
0.5	29
1.0	50
2.0	75
3.0	88
3.3	**90**
4.0	94
5.0	97
7.0	99

Figure 1.10 Percentage of steady state level reached at various times after initiating or changing drug therapy. The minimum time after which reliable steady state measurements can be made is emphasised.

It is frequently stated that five half-lives must elapse before plateau concentrations are achieved, unless loading doses are employed when they are attained much more rapidly. It will be seen from Figure 1.10 that the plasma concentration after 3.3 half-lives is 90% of the predicted steady state and this may be taken as the minimum time for sampling after starting the drug or changing the dose. For drugs with a long half-life (e.g. digoxin, phenobarbitone), two weeks or more may be required before steady state samples can be taken, especially if renal function is poor and the drug is renally excreted (e.g. digoxin).

It should be noted that in the neonate, the rapidly changing clinical state, degree of hydration and dosage requirements make the idea of steady state a theoretical concept rather than an attainable goal in many cases, and there is little value in delaying concentration measurements for such a hypothetical steady state to be established. In unstable situations where attainment of steady state is subject to variable absorption, distribution or excretion the administration of a loading dose effectively achieves steady state; this enables sampling to be undertaken thereafter. Data obtained in such a situation will require particularly careful interpretation.

A further requirement for many drugs is to take samples at the appropriate time following the last dose. Serum digoxin concentrations do not reflect tissue concentrations for at least six hours following dosing due to continuing distribution, and specimens for digoxin analysis should not be taken during this period. Contrary to a frequently expressed belief, this requirement is not negated by intravenous dosing, as there is still a considerable distribution period before the drug reaches equilibrium between the plasma space and the tissue compartment containing the receptor. Further details for individual drugs are given in Chapter 2.

The size of the fluctuations in plasma concentration between doses obviously depends on the dosage interval and the plasma half-life. Frequent dosing avoids large peaks and transient toxic effects, but is unpopular with patients, difficult to comply with and more likely to lead to medication errors. Less frequent dosing gives rise to large fluctuations in concentration. To some extent, these opposing considerations can be reconciled with the use of sustained release preparations.

There is no single optimum time for taking samples in relation to dose. The most reproducible time to take measurements is immediately pre-dose (trough concentration), when the lowest concentrations in the cycle will be obtained. This is best if an indication of drug efficacy is required, and will show least between-sample variability in patients on chronic therapy. The use of peak and trough concentrations for detecting toxicity of aminoglycoside antibiotics has become less relevant with once-daily dosing regimens, but sampling at two hours post dose for ciclosporin has become a common and effective TDM technique. This type of sampling in the absorption/distribution phase is highly sensitive to accurate determination of sampling time in relation to dose. The average steady state concentration may be obtained by taking samples approximately midway between doses.

When computer programs are used for pharmacokinetic parameter optimisation and dosage prediction (see Chapter 4), it becomes extremely important that dosage and sampling times are accurately known, as large prediction errors can result from poor data.

Accurate analysis
This requirement will be considered as part of the analytical section in Chapter 3.

Interpretation
Even if a relevant question has been formulated, an appropriate specimen taken and an accurate result obtained, the whole exercise is valueless unless the result is correctly interpreted and any necessary action taken. Interpretation of drug concentrations requires knowledge of the pharmacokinetic and pharmacodynamic factors outlined earlier, and may demand considerable expertise. Unfortunately, without effective education programmes, users of TDM services frequently interpret results simply by comparing them with the target range and then either do nothing or react to bring the concentrations closer to the quoted range. Much harm can be done by this process, since it is frequently forgotten by

clinicians, as well as laboratory workers, that the aim of the TDM process is to ameliorate the patient's symptoms rather than to get drug concentrations into a particular range.

The target range is a combination of two concepts – the minimum effective concentration for a drug and the maximum safe concentration. Between these limits, the majority of patients should experience maximum therapeutic benefit at minimal risk of toxicity and undesirable side effects. However, this simple theory breaks down in a number of important respects, and the target range must always be considered as an adjunct to clinical judgement and not a substitute for it. For this reason, the term *target range* is preferred over the older term 'therapeutic range'. It can be argued that the lower limit of the target range should be abandoned altogether, since response to a drug is a continuum, and some patients do show a significant response at apparently 'sub-therapeutic' concentrations.

In Shorvon and Reynolds' early work on controlling newly diagnosed epileptic patients on a single anticonvulsant, a quarter of the patients could be controlled on carbamazepine or phenytoin at concentrations below the target range. Similarly, many epileptic patients require concentrations well in excess of the normally accepted range to control their fits. Such patients are often untroubled by symptoms of toxicity, and will experience further seizures if the dose of drug is reduced.

The optimum range of drug concentrations for a particular patient is a very individual matter, depending to some extent on the severity of the underlying disease process. This fact does not undermine the value of TDM, but does require a clear understanding of why an individual request has been ordered and how it can be interpreted in the light of the patient's condition. There is no reason to monitor drug concentrations in a patient who is clinically stable and not showing symptoms of toxicity, except perhaps on one occasion as a baseline in case problems are subsequently encountered.

Difficulties arise when, having made a measurement for no particularly good reason in a stable patient, the clinician discovers that the result is outside the target range and feels compelled to do something about it. It must be said that this is sometimes provoked by laboratory workers, some of whom label all results above the target range as 'toxic', and telephone them in alarmed tones. In one of the earliest papers on TDM, Koch-Weser wrote: "Therapeutic decisions should never be based solely on the drug concentration in the serum". The cardinal principle, often repeated but still forgotten, is to *treat the patient rather than the drug concentration.*

Response

Drug concentrations above the target range do not invariably require a reduction in dosage. For immunosuppresants it may be necessary in some patients to maintain concentrations above the target range to avoid rejection of transplanted organs. For other drugs it may be that if the patient is symptom-free, a careful search for signs of toxicity should be made. If no evidence is found, the patient may be best served by doing nothing, although for some drugs (e.g. phenytoin) continued monitoring for the development of long-term undesirable effects is advisable. Similarly, drug concentrations below the target range in a patient who is well and free from symptoms do not require an increased dose, although in some cases (e.g. digoxin) they may provide evidence that the drug is no longer necessary and stopping it under medical supervision is worth trying.

Organisation of a TDM service – who and where?

The basic essentials for an effective TDM service are the availability of appropriate analytical methods, specialist expertise and the ability to produce results within a clinically relevant time. The analytical aspects of these requirements will be discussed in detail in Chapter 3, but some discussion of the specialist expertise required and what constitutes a clinically relevant turn-round time is now required.

Staff

An effective TDM service requires experienced analysts who understand the basis of the procedures involved and are competent to advise on the analytical sensitivity and specificity of the methods in use and to maintain exacting standards of accuracy and precision. In addition, it is essential that the service has access to a source of specialist advice on interpretation from someone who understands pharmacokinetics and therapeutics. Whether this expertise resides with the clinician, the pharmacist or the laboratory scientist is less important than the fact that it exists somewhere and can be accessed when required. For routine service provision, laboratory staff are likely to be best placed to maintain a service across a range of clinical situations.

The best service is generally obtained with a team approach in which pharmacists, clinical biochemists, technical and medical staff all play a role. The specialist staff involved may act in various ways. The most effective way to make good use of a TDM service in difficult cases is for TDM requests to be discussed with one of the clinical leads e.g. a clinical pharmacist, before any samples are taken. They can advise on whether the request is indicated, and on the appropriate timing of any samples required. Following analysis, results are scrutinised by members of the team and appropriate recommendations for action conveyed to the clinician.

However, this ideal degree of involvement is impractical for many hospitals due to staffing constraints or lack of available expertise and becomes even more difficult in out-patient or primary care work. To gain most from a request it is essential that the request form contains full information on the reason for analysis, dosage regime, length of time on therapy, the time of the specimen in relation to the last dose, other prescribed drugs and the clinical status of the patient. If the specimen or the reason for analysis is inappropriate, specialist laboratory staff can then contact the clinician and suggest a course of action; regrettably such information is provided infrequently.

Intervention after the analysis has been performed is obviously less effective in controlling the number of inappropriate requests, but nonetheless has a role in improving the use that is made of TDM services. All results, or just those which fall outside defined limits, can be followed up by specialist staff who are able to evaluate their significance and make appropriate recommendations to the requesting doctor. However, it must be stressed that informed opinion is still required at this stage of intervention. The practice in some laboratories of simply glancing at the result and commenting 'toxic' if it is above the target range or 'sub-therapeutic' if it is below it, almost certainly does more harm than good (as with all unthinking comments on reports!).

Turnround time and point-of care-testing
As with all point-of-care-testing (POCT) the key question to be addressed is 'why is the result required immediately'? However, there are currently no acceptable devices for POCT for quantitative TDM. In routine practice there is little clinical need for analyses to be performed on the spot, provided that a local service is available which can produce results within a matter of hours if appropriate transport arrangements can be made.

POCT devices have been available for TDM in the past, and have been shown to have a positive impact on the efficiency of out-patient clinics for asthma and anti-convulsant monitoring in an epilepsy clinic. While the devices used are no longer available there may be a case for out-patient clinics with a large proportion of patients requiring TDM being sited close to a rapid-response laboratory or linked by pneumatic tube or other rapid transport arrangements.

The provision of a near-patient service is often expensive in staff time and also in reagent costs, since the need for a rapid result generally necessitates the use of more expensive immunoassay systems, although portable HPLC systems have been used.

Effectiveness of TDM – does it help patients?

In an era of evidence-based medicine the lack of early studies into the efficacy of TDM has undermined its informed use. The studies that have accompanied the development and effective utilisation of immunosuppressants and more recent studies on aminoglycosides have proved that properly applied TDM is effective and that the consequences of not performing adequate TDM for this class of drugs are dire. The lesser impact in other areas of TDM emphasizes the need for clinical judgement for effective application, rather than uncritical ticking of boxes.

In some surveys, two thirds or more of requests made to TDM services have been shown to be inadequately thought out, badly executed or misinterpreted. Requesting clinicians are frequently unclear as to when TDM would be helpful, and reluctant to pay proper attention to the results once obtained. The consequence of this has been an increasing workload for analytical laboratories and considerable wastage of analytical and financial resources, plus diminished standards of patient care and an understandable degree of cynicism about the whole process. It is now clear that the availability of accurate TDM data does not in itself improve symptom control or reduce the incidence of toxicity in themselves. As long ago as 1985, in an editorial on TDM, the Lancet noted, "If plasma drug assays are to be done, they must be accompanied by some form of education system that tells the prescribing doctor the meaning of the result and what steps should now be taken." This statement remains as true today as it was when it was written.

Experience has shown that attempts to educate general users of TDM services have very limited effect except in the case of specialist services e.g. transplantation. The availability of Intranet or Internet information linked to results reporting systems does, however, hold out the prospect of providing targeted information at the moment that it is required, and enabling more informed use of TDM data.

Further reading

Baastrup PC, Schou M. Lithium as a prophylactic agent. Arch Gen Psychiatr 1967; **16:** 162-172.

Binder L, Schiel X, Binder C, et al. Clinical outcome and economic impact of aminoglycoside peak concentrations in febrile immunocompromised patients with haematological malignancies. Clin Chem 1998; **44:** 408-14.

Brodie MJ. The optimum use of anticonvulsants. Practitioner 1985; **229:** 921-927.

Buchthal F, Svensmark O, Schiller PJ. Clinical and electroencephalographic correlations with serum levels of diphenylhydantoin. Arch Neurol 1960; **2:** 624-631.

Editorial. What therapeutic drugs should be monitored? Lancet 1985; **II:** 309-310.

Elliot K, Watson ID, Tsintis P et al. The impact of near-patient testing on the organisation and costs of an anticonvulsant clinic. Ther Drug Monit 1990; **12:** 434-437.

Hallworth MJ. Audit of therapeutic drug monitoring. Ann Clin Biochem 1988; **25:** 121-128.

Houtman PN, Hall SK, Green A, Rylance GW. Rapid anticonvulsant monitoring in an epilepsy clinic. Arch Dis Child 1990; **65:** 264-268.

Koch-Weser J. Drug therapy: serum drug concentrations as therapeutic guides. N Engl J Med 1972; **287:** 227-231.

Marshall EK Jr, Dearborn EH. The relation of the plasma concentration of quinacrine to its antimalarial activity. J Pharmacol Exp Ther 1946; **88:** 142-153.

Schumacher GE, Barr JT. Total testing process applied to therapeutic drug monitoring: impact on patients' outcomes and economics. Clin Chem 1998; **44:** 370-4.

Shorvon SD, Reynolds EH. Early prognosis of epilepsy. Br Med J 1982; **285:** 1699-1701.

Spector R, Park GD, Johnson GF, Vesell ES. Therapeutic Drug Monitoring. Clin Pharm Ther 1988; **43:** 345-353.

Watson ID. Clinical Drug Testing at the Point of Care. In: Price CP, St John A, Hicks JM (eds) Point of Care Testing. Washington DC: AACC Press, 2nd Edn 2004: 435-443.

Chapter 2

Individual drugs

ANTIBIOTICS

Aminoglycosides (gentamicin, tobramycin, amikacin and netilmicin)

Clinical use

The aminoglycosides are an important group of antimicrobial drugs used in the treatment of severe systemic infection by some Gram-positive and many Gram-negative organisms. Amikacin, gentamicin and tobramycin are also active against *Pseudomonas aeruginosa*. Streptomycin is active against *Mycobacterium tuberculosis* and is now generally reserved for tuberculosis.

The parent compounds are produced by moulds of the *Streptomyces* family (strep-tomycin, tobramycin and neomycin) or the *Micromonospora* family (gentamicin and netilmicin). The different host organisms account for the variation in spelling of the suffix. Aminoglycosides interfere with protein synthesis in susceptible microorganisms. Although most inhibitors of microbial protein synthesis are bacteriostatic, the aminoglycosides are also bacteriocidal. Neomycin is too toxic for systemic use.

Pharmacokinetics

The aminoglycoside antibiotics exhibit relatively simple pharmacokinetics.

IMPORTANT FACTS

- Large, highly polar molecules
- Very poor oral bioavailability – must be given parenterally
- Not plasma protein bound
- Not metabolised
- Excreted renally
- Short plasma half-life (2 - 3 h), except when renal function impaired

The terminal phase of gentamicin elimination has an extremely long half-life, as the drug becomes concentrated in tissues, and elimination from these sites is very slow. If therapy is continued for longer than a week, tissue sites become saturated and plasma concentrations may rise.

There are marked intra-individual variations in the rate of absorption from an intramuscular dose, volume of distribution and plasma half-life (dependent on renal function), which means that the relationship between dose and concentration is poor.

SUMMARY OF AMINOGLYCOSIDE PHARMACOKINETICS

Parameter	Gentamicin	Amikacin
Oral bioavailability (F)	<0.05	<0.05
Fraction excreted renally	>0.9	0.98
Fraction bound to plasma proteins	<0.1	<0.1
Clearance (corrected for bioavailability) (mL/min/kg)*	1.0 - 1.5	1.0 - 1.5
Volume of distribution V_d (L/kg)	0.18 - 0.52	0.14 - 0.36
Elimination half-life (h) *	2-3	2-3
Time to maximum concentration (h) (im)	1	1
Parameter	Netilmicin	Tobramycin
Oral bioavailability (F)	<0.05	<0.05
Fraction excreted renally	0.8 - 0.9	0.9
Fraction bound to plasma proteins	<0.1	<0.1
Clearance (corrected for bioavailability) (mL/min/kg)*	1.0 - 1.5	1.0 - 1.5
Volume of distribution V_d (L/Kg)	0.2	0.1 - 0.3
Elimination half-life (h) *	2 - 3	2 - 3
Time to maximum concentration (h) (im/iv)	1	1

* if renal function unimpaired

Toxicity

Antimicrobial drugs normally have a high therapeutic index, and supratherapeutic doses may be given safely (e.g. penicillins, macrolides, sulfonamides). The situation is different for aminoglycosides, where significant toxicity may occur just above the plasma concentration required for bactericidal activity. Aminoglycosides are carried into bacteria by active transport, but some mammalian cells (notably the renal tubular cell and the auditory hair cell) also possess this transport mechanism.

IMPORTANT FACTS

- Main toxic effects are nephrotoxicity and ototoxicity
- Nephrotoxicity further reduces aminoglycoside excretion, precipitating a vicious cycle
- Nephrotoxicity is usually reversible
- Mild ototoxicity is also reversible, but severely damaged hair cells cannot be replaced and patients may be left with irreversible hearing loss and disturbed equilibrium

Clinical use of aminoglycosides is a delicate balance between achieving the concentrations necessary for effect and avoiding toxicity. Failure to achieve adequate concentrations can result in treatment failure and the development of antibiotic resistance. Therapeutic drug monitoring is vital in achieving effective therapy.

Monitoring therapy
The drug concentration at which bacteriocidal effects are achieved (the minimum inhibitory concentration, MIC) is relatively easy to measure *in vitro*, but often has little relevance *in vivo*, due to variable penetration of the drug to the site of infection and differing conditions at the infection site. Furthermore, aminoglycosides show a marked post-antibiotic effect – suppression of bacterial growth persists for some time after the antibiotic is no longer present in the plasma. Definition of therapeutic ranges is therefore extremely difficult, and this difficulty has been compounded recently by changes in the ways in which aminoglycoside antibiotics have been administered.

Aminoglycosides have been used widely in clinical practice for over 30 years, and for most of that time established practice was to give them in two or three divided doses. It has become clear that once daily dosing produces higher peak concentrations (enhancing the bacterial kill) and lower trough concentrations (reducing the risk of toxicity). Such regimes are more convenient, reduce adaptive resistance and are often more suitable in patients with normal renal function.

The approach was originally devised as once daily dosing, but a more accurate term is probably 'extended dosing interval', in which a plasma concentration measurement is used to design a dosing interval which reflects the needs of the individual patient (particularly taking into account renal function). Such an approach is exemplified by the Hartford nomogram for determining the repeat dosing interval of gentamicin given in a standard dose of 7 mg/kg (Nicolau *et al.*, 1995) – see Chapter 4. Various other schemes have been described. Extended dose regimes are generally not suitable for children, pregnant or breast feeding women and patients with ascites, endocarditis, cystic fibrosis, serious burns, neutropenia or severe renal failure.

These strategies have posed challenges to therapeutic drug monitoring services, and assays in many cases have not had sufficient sensitivity to measure the concentrations found at 24 - 48 hours post dose. Guidelines as to doses and plasma concentrations on extended-dose regimes remain controversial, and expert advice should be sought for specific regimes.

For conventional (divided-dose) regimes, trough concentrations and peak (1 h post-dose [im or iv]) concentrations should be:

		Trough (mg/L)	Peak (mg/L)
Gentamicin	)	< 2	5 - 10
Tobramycin	)	(< 1 in endocarditis)	(3 - 5 in endocarditis)
Netilmicin	)		
Amikacin		< 10	20 - 30

Molar units are not used for aminoglycoside assays as the precise composition of the molecular species administered is unknown.

Monitoring should be undertaken in all patients after the 2nd - 4th dose, earlier if renal function is poor or changing or if other risk factors for toxicity are present. Monitoring is **essential** in infants, the elderly, in obesity, in cystic fibrosis, if high doses are being used or if renal function is impaired.

Glycopeptides (vancomycin and teicoplanin)

Clinical Use
Vancomycin and teicoplanin have antibiotic activity against aerobic and anaerobic Gram-positive bacteria. Vancomycin is given intravenously (oral absorption is poor) in the prophylaxis and treatment of endocarditis and other serious infections caused by Gram-positive cocci, including multi-resistant cocci, notably multi-resistant *Staphylococcus aureus* (MRSA). It has a relatively long duration of action and can be given every 12 hours. Teicoplanin is very similar to vancomycin, but has a longer duration of action allowing once daily administration. It can be given intramuscularly as well as intravenously.

Pharmacokinetics

Like the aminoglycosides, glycopeptides are poorly absorbed and renally excreted.

SUMMARY OF VANCOMYCIN PHARMACOKINETICS

Parameter	Vancomycin
Oral bioavailability (F)	<0.05
Fraction excreted renally	0.8
Fraction bound to plasma proteins	0.2 - 0.4
Clearance (corrected for bioavailability) (mL/min/kg)	1.0 - 1.5
Volume of distribution V_d (L/kg)	0.3 - 0.5
Elimination half-life (h)	4 - 6
Time to maximum concentration (h)	<1

Toxicity

As for the aminoglycosides, nephrotoxicity and ototoxicity may occur at plasma concentrations above therapeutic concentrations. The risk of toxicity is enhanced if aminoglycosides are given concurrently. The most common adverse reaction, flushing of the upper body ('red man' syndrome) occurs if the drug is infused too rapidly or too high a plasma concentration is attained. Discontinuing the infusion results in resolution of the clinical features of toxicity.

Monitoring therapy

Considerable controversy has surrounded the question of whether concentration monitoring of glycopeptides is worthwhile, but recent studies support a role for monitoring in ensuring maximum effect with minimum toxicity. Some workers support monitoring in all patient groups treated for > 48 hours, while others feel it is worthwhile only in clinically defined sub-groups at high risk, such as those receiving other nephrotoxic drugs or with pre-existing renal impairment, children and pregnant patients.

Increasing the concentration of vancomycin within the target range does not decrease the time taken to kill the bacterial population, so there is scant evidence for a concentration-effect relationship within the target range. Vancomycin also exhibits a post-antibiotic effect.

Effective plasma concentrations are usually taken to be 20 - 40 mg/L (peak [1 h]) and 5 - 10 mg/L (trough) for vancomycin. For teicoplanin, suggested target ranges are 20 - 60 mg/L for *Staphylococcus aureus* and 10 - 60 mg/L in other infections (pre-dose samples).

Other antibiotics/antifungals

Chloramphenicol is a powerful broad spectrum antibiotic that is associated with serious haematological side effects when given systemically. It is used to treat life-threatening infections such as cholera, typhoid fever and resistant *Haemophilus influenzae*, septicaemia and meningitis. It is metabolised in the liver to the inactive glucuronide and the metabolite (and some parent drug) is excreted renally. Over a 24h period, 75-90% of an administered dose appears in the urine, about 5-10% in the biologically active form.

Plasma concentrations between 10 - 25 mg/L (30 - 77 µmol/L) are desirable. Myelosuppression is seen most commonly with sustained plasma concentrations above 25 mg/L (77 µmol/L). Monitoring is essential in neonates and desirable in children under four, the elderly and patients with hepatic impairment.

Sulfamethoxazole and trimethoprim (co-trimoxazole) when used in high dosage (for example against *Pneumocystitis carinii*), the antituberculous agent cicloserine and the antifungal flucytosine may also require monitoring, especially in patients with renal impairment.

Structures of some antibiotics

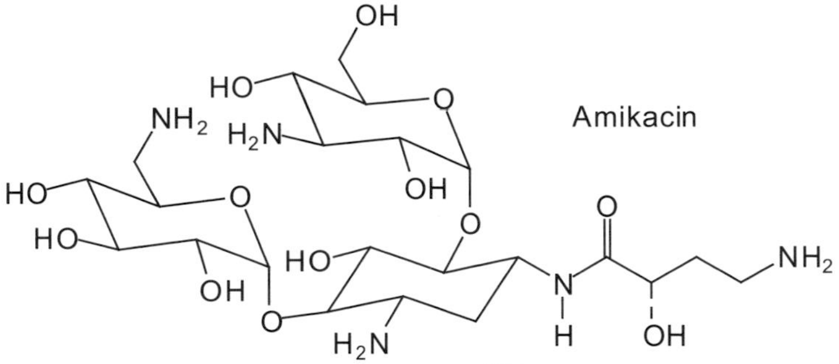

Amikacin

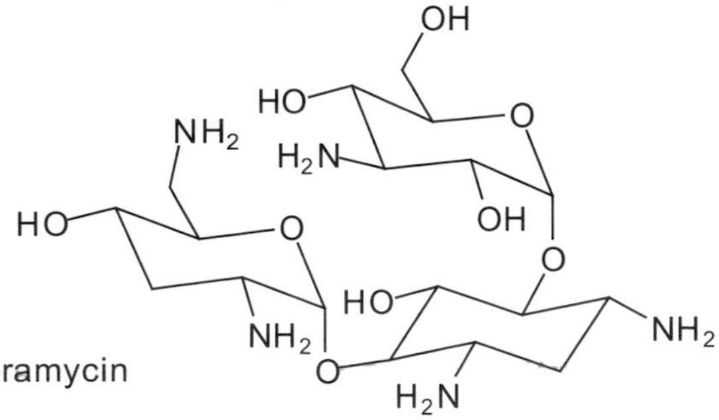

Tobramycin

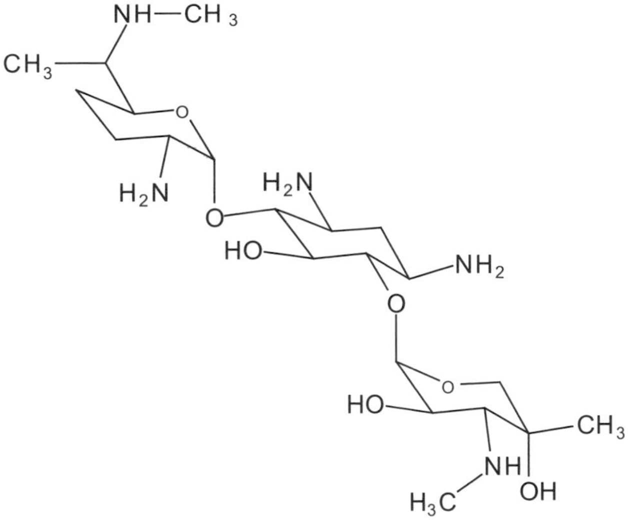

Gentamicin

ANTI-CANCER DRUGS

Methotrexate

Clinical Use

IMPORTANT FACTS

- Reduces the C1 pool, causing reduction in folate availability
- Inhibits dihydrofolate reductase
- Effective in psoriasis, rheumatoid arthritis and other autoimmune diseases

Methotrexate (MTX) has a unique place in chemotherapy. It was the first agent to effect a cure of a cancer – choriocarcinoma. The depletion of the carbon 1 pool due to inhibition of dihydrofolate reductase (DHFR) reduces folate availability, disrupting purine synthesis. It is effective in the treatment of childhood leukaemias, but not in adult leukaemias. In high doses MTX has been shown to be effective in osteosarcoma, but there is a need for folate rescue using leucovorin. MTX is also effective in combination with other anti-neoplastic agents. The lipophobic nature of MTX necessitates intrathecal introduction to challenge any CNS tumour, typically leukaemia. The lower doses used to treat rheumatoid arthritis or psoriasis do not usually result in the need for leucovorin rescue and routine monitoring is not required.

Resistance to MTX can occur via a number of mechanisms: impaired cellular MTX uptake, increased DHFR activity, impaired DHFR recognition of MTX and changes in MTX metabolism. These mechanisms may arise through selection of cell lines during therapy, with vulnerable tumour cell lines being affected allowing the resistant clone to remain viable.

Pharmacokinetics

IMPORTANT FACTS

- ~90% excreted unchanged renally
- Some biliary excretion
- High doses result in metabolites e.g. 7-hydroxy MTX
- Polyglutamate metabolites accumulate intracellularly

There is complete absorption of the oral doses of MTX used in non-cancer applications e.g. psoriasis or rheumatoid arthritis. The higher doses required for chemotherapy need to be given intravenously.

MTX exhibits a triphasic elimination profile: the initial phase reflects distribution, the next phase renal elimination and the final phase elimination from intracellular distribution. This may be prolonged in the presence of renal failure or ascites. As the mode of action of MTX depends on C1 depletion toxicity affects rapidly dividing cells such as bone marrow and higher concentrations perpetuate toxic effects. Alkalinisation improves renal clearance and minimises MTX nephrotoxicity.

SUMMARY OF METHOTREXATE PHARMACOKINETICS

Parameter	Methotrexate
Oral bioavailability (F)	~ 0.7 low dose ~ 0.2 high dose*
Fraction excreted renally	<0.9
Fraction bound to plasma proteins	~ 0.5
Clearance (corrected for bioavailability) (mL/min/kg)	2.0 - 3.0
Volume of distribution V_d (L/kg)	0.35 - 0.75
Elimination half-life (h)	5 - 9
Time to maximum concentration (h) dose	~ 1.0 po low

Toxicity

IMPORTANT FACTS

- Kills rapidly dividing cells e.g. bone marrow
- Renal impairment exacerbates toxicity
- Chronic low dose use can cause cirrhosis
- Chronic low dose use may cause reversible increases in plasma aminotransferase activity
- High plasma concentrations > 450 µg/L (**1 µmol/L** NB: methotrexate concentrations are conventionally expressed in molar units) after 48 hours require high dose leucovorin rescue

MTX acute toxicity is due to death of cells with rapid turnover e.g. GI epithelia. Low dose toxicity is cumulative in susceptible patients resulting in portal fibrosis and cirrhosis; changes in plasma aminotransferases are reversible. There is a risk of spontaneous haemorrhage. Bone marrow depletion leaves the patient open to potentially fatal infection. MTX causes nephrotoxicity when given in high dose. This appears to be related to solubility in acidic urine and is addressed by pre-alkalinisation of the urine prior to dosing. MTX causes neurotoxicity when given intrathecally. Malignant effusions can become a reservoir for MTX resulting in continued slow elimination and consequently toxicity. Haemodialysis can assist in removing MTX in these circumstances.

Monitoring Therapy

IMPORTANT FACTS

- Measurement 48 hours post-dose to confirm plasma MTX concentration is < 450 µg/L (**1 µmol/L**)
- If above this threshold, monitor concentrations to below the toxic concentration of 9 µg/L (**20 nmol/L**)
- Monitor full blood count in low dose patients to detect thrombocytopenia

Structure of methotrexate

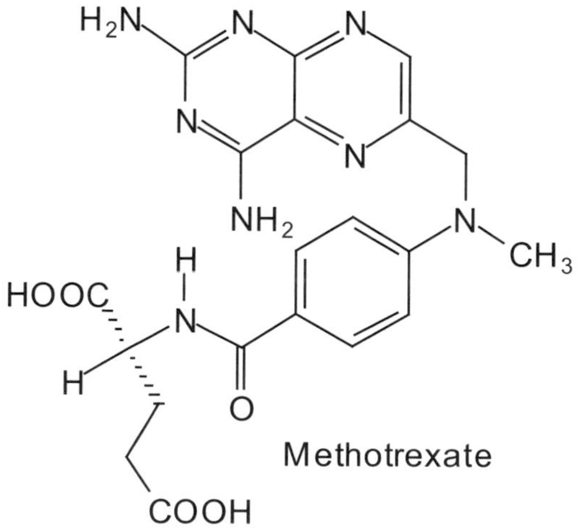

Methotrexate

ANTICONVULSANTS

Carbamazepine

Clinical use

IMPORTANT FACTS:

- Widely used anticonvulsant
- Used in bipolar affective disorder, mania and depression as a mood stabilizer
- Effective in trigeminal neuralgia

Carbamazepine (CBZ: Tegretol, Novartis) is one of the drugs of choice for the treatment of generalised tonic-clonic (grand mal) and partial (focal) seizures. Carbamazepine inhibits voltage-gated fast sodium channels, and exerts a stabilising effect on excitable membranes. The anticonvulsant action is thought to be due to inhibition of high frequency discharges from seizure foci and reduction of the spread of neuronal excitation, although (as is the case for all anticonvulsants) the details are not well understood. For generalised tonic-clonic seizures there is little difference between CBZ, phenytoin and sodium valproate as far as efficacy is concerned, and the eventual choice is often the best tolerated drug. Partial epilepsy is more difficult to control, and either CBZ or phenytoin is the traditional first-line choice for both simple and complex seizures. CBZ is not indicated for absence (petit mal) attacks.

Carbamazepine is an accepted therapy for the treatment of bipolar disease and is effective in ~ 60% patients with manic and depressive symptoms. Carbamazepine is also used for the treatment of trigeminal neuralgia and diabetic neuropathy. Its antidiuretic effect has been employed in the treatment of diabetes insipidus.

Pharmacokinetics

IMPORTANT FACTS

- Metabolised to the epoxide then the dihydrodiol by CYP3A4 and CYP2C8
- Induces its own metabolism
- Metabolism is induced by phenobarbital and phenytoin
- Metabolism inhibited by valproate and lamotrigine

Around 75% of a dose is absorbed from the gut. CBZ is metabolised in the liver by the cytochrome P450 isoenzymes CYP3A4 and CYP2C8 to form the predominant metabolite carbamazepine-10,11-epoxide (CBZ-E) (Figure 2.1), which has comparable anticonvulsant activity to the parent drug. The epoxide is further metabolised to carbamazepine-10,11-dihydrodiol. CBZ has a plasma half-life of between 5-30 hours, the lower value reflects induction of its own metabolism, which occurs on chronic administration; the epoxide has a plasma half-life of around 5 hours. Towards the end of the first month of therapy, plasma concentrations fall by about 25% and the dose may need to be increased to maintain the anticonvulsant effect. Metabolism is also induced by other anticonvulsants, notably phenobarbitone and phenytoin. Metabolism of CBZ-E is inhibited by valproate and lamotrigine, resulting in a doubling of CBZ-E concentrations at constant dose.The extensive metabolism of CBZ means that loss of renal function does not cause accumulation.

SUMMARY OF CARBAMAZEPINE PHARMACOKINETICS

Parameter	Carbamazepine
Oral bioavailability (F)	0.75
Fraction excreted renally	< 0.01
Fraction bound to plasma proteins	~ 0.75
Clearance (corrected for bioavailability) (mL/min/kg)	0.8 - 1.8
Volume of distribution V_d (L/Kg)	1.0 - 1.8
Elimination half-life (h)	10 - 20
Time to maximum concentration Tmax (h)	4 - 8

Toxicity

IMPORTANT FACTS

- Dose limiting side effects: blurred vision, dizziness, ataxia
- Erythematous rash in 3 - 5% of patients
- Syndrome of inappropriate antidiuresis may occur
- Rarely leucopenia

Carbamazepine has fewer side effects than phenytoin or phenobarbital, but reversible blurring of vision, dizziness and unsteadiness may be dose limiting. The neurotoxic effects appear to be related to peak plasma concentrations, and may be minimised by altering the dosage regime or using a controlled-release formulation. A generalised erythematous rash may occur in 3 -5% of patients. The drug is particularly free of long-term side effects, but hyponatraemia due to inappropriate antidiuresis occurs and cardiac failure may occur as a late complication, especially in the elderly. Serious haematological toxicity (notably leucopenia and agranulocytosis) has also been reported.

Carbamazepine metabolism

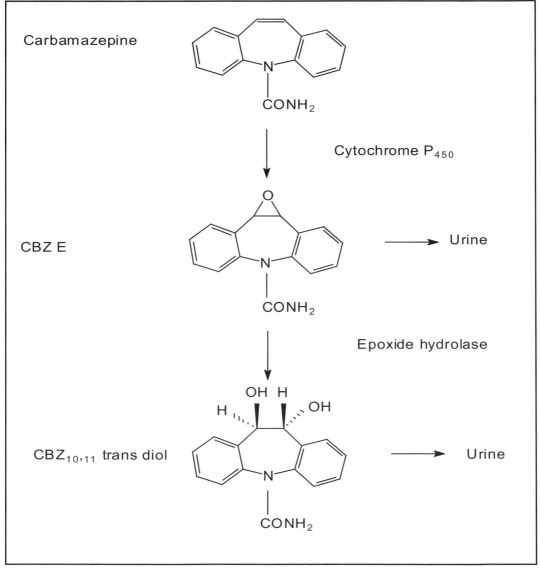

Figure 2.1 Formation and elimination of carbamazepine 10,11 - epoxide (CBZ E)

Monitoring therapy

- Typical target range: 4 - 12 mg/L (17 - 50 µmol/L)
- The epoxide metabolite is pharmacologically active
- The epoxide is rarely measured, but should be
- Trough plasma concentration is a better guide to therapy than dose

The relationship between trough plasma CBZ concentration and clinical response is complicated by the presence of an active metabolite and by individual pharmacodynamic variability. A lower limit of the target range is difficult to define. Some patients undoubtedly show a response at concentrations below 4 mg/L (17 µmol/L), but maximum therapeutic benefit usually requires concentrations above 6 mg/L (25 µmol/L). Some patients (particularly those with complex partial epilepsy) may require concentrations above 12 mg/L (50 µmol/L) for optimum anticonvulsant effect, and in such situations the degree of clinical response may be limited by the development of unacceptable neurotoxicity. Dizziness and visual disturbances become increasingly frequent at plasma concentrations above 10 mg/L (42 µmol/L). Side effects may occur at lower CBZ concentrations in patients on combination therapy.

Since dosage of CBZ is a poor guide to plasma concentration, therapeutic drug monitoring is necessary when seizure control is difficult to obtain. Some patients can be managed effectively with minimal monitoring, as the relationship between dose and plasma concentration in the individual patient is linear once the phase of metabolic induction is complete. A baseline concentration measurement when seizures are effectively controlled is useful, in case compliance problems or pharmacokinetic changes (e.g. in pregnancy or acute illness) cause difficulties subsequently.

As CBZ concentrations can vary quite markedly across the dosage interval (especially once induction has resulted in more rapid clearance), isolated measurements can be difficult to interpret, and standardisation of sample timing is advisable for long-term monitoring. Trough measurements are the most reproducible. It would be unusual to measure concentrations at any other time unless there are specific issues in an individual patient.

Ethosuximide

Clinical Uses

IMPORTANT FACTS

- Used in absence seizure
- Not used in tonic-clonic seizure
- Of minor interest

Principally used in paediatric absence seizures. The mode of action is to reduce thalamic calcium current thresholds. It is not effective in tonic-clonic seizure.

Pharmacokinetics

IMPORTANT FACTS

- Metabolised to inactive hydroxyethyl metabolite
- Poorly protein bound

Ethosuximide is a chiral drug, but used clinically as a racemate. Absorption peak concentrations occur around 3 hours with a volume of distribution of 0.7 L/kg; the major metabolite is the inactive hydroxyethyl metabolite through CYP3A4 metabolism. Around 20% of the dose is excreted unchanged in urine. The half-life in children is approximately 30 hours; adults is twice as long. Ethosuximide is poorly protein bound.

SUMMARY OF ETHOSUXIMIDE PHARMACOKINETICS

Parameter	Ethosuximide
Oral bioavailability (F)	0.95
Fraction excreted renally	0.2
Fraction bound to plasma proteins	<0.05
Clearance (corrected for bioavailability) (mL/min/kg)	0.15-0.22
Volume of distribution V_d (L/kg)	0.6-0.8
Elimination half-life (h)	40-60
Time to maximum concentration (h)	2-4 (adults) 3-7 (children)

Toxicity

IMPORTANT FACTS

- GI disturbances
- CNS disturbances

Gastrointestinal disturbances are most common and CNS disturbances such as dizziness, lethargy occurs but tolerance develops to these.

Monitoring therapy

IMPORTANT FACTS

- Change dose slowly
- Monitoring rarely necessary

A target range of 40-100 μg/L (280-700 μmol/L) is quoted. The long half-life requires slow dose changes and dosing should be incremented on commencing therapy. The occurrence of potential symptoms of toxicity might be considered a reason for plasma concentration measurement, but is rarely necessary. Haematopoietic and dermal side-effects may occur.

Felbamate

Clinical use

IMPORTANT FACTS

- Adjunct therapy in epilepsy
- Effective in Lennox-Gastaut Syndrome

Currently used as an adjunct in therapy of partial seizures, it can be effective in patients refractory to other treatments, perhaps related to its selective effect on ictal patterns. It has been particularly successful in the treatment of Lennox-Gastaut Syndrome, a childhood disorder characterised by multiple seizures, slow spike-wave electroencephalograms and mental retardation; hitherto it was resistant to drug therapy. However, felbamate has a significant incidence of dose related side effects and idiosyncratic reactions that limit its acceptance as a first-line treatment. Felbamate enhances the efficacy of the GABA system and also inhibits excitatory amino acid responses. It is thought to interact with N-methyl-

D-aspartate (NMDA) receptors.

Pharmacokinetics

Important facts

- Metabolised by CYP3A4 and CYP2E1
- Phenytoin and carbamazepine increase clearance

Felbamate is well absorbed following oral dosing (~ 90%), though children (4 - 12 years) demonstrate a dose proportionality. Around 25% is bound to albumin, 50% is excreted unchanged in urine, the remainder is metabolised by the cytochrome P450 isoenzymes CYP3A4 and CYP2E1. Not all metabolites have been characterised, but they include the non-pharmacologically active: 2-hydroxyfelbamate, para-hydroxyfelbamate and felbamate monocarbamate.

Felbamate inhibits CYP2C19 and hence affects carbamazepine 10,11 epoxide clearance; there is a similar affect on phenytoin. Paradoxically due to induction of CYP3A4 the clearance of carbamazepine itself is induced, both it and its 10,11 epoxide are pharmacologically active. Carbamazepine, phenytoin and phenobarbital all induce felbamate clearance.

Summary of felbamate pharmacokinetics

Parameter	Felbamate
Oral bioavailability (F)	> 0.9
Fraction excreted renally	~ 0.5
Fraction bound to plasma proteins	~ 0.25
Clearance (corrected for bioavailability) (mL/min/kg)	0.4 - 0.6
Volume of distribution V_d (L/kg)	~ 0.8
Elimination half-life (h)	~ 20
Time to maximum concentration (h)	1 - 4

Toxicity

IMPORTANT FACTS

- Risk of serious toxicity: aplastic anaemia; hepatic failure
- Toxicity limits restricts use to intractable epilepsy

Common side effects include: anorexia, weight loss, nausea, vomiting, insomnia, headache, dizziness and somnolence. However, there are two serious side effects: aplastic anaemia and hepatic failure. The development of aplastic anaemia has been attributed to a reactive metabolite, atropaldehyde; susceptilibity may be linked to deficient glutathione peroxidase, superoxide dismutase or glutathione reductase activity. This risk of toxicity means that felbamate is reserved for patients with epilepsy that is difficult to control with other drugs.

Monitoring therapy

IMPORTANT FACTS

- Monitor liver function tests and full blood counts
- Increases phenytoin, phenobarbitone and valproate concentrations
- Decreases carbamazepine concentrations

Due to the risk of toxicity, regular (< 4 weekly) monitoring of liver function tests and full blood counts are essential. Therapy is initiated slowly and incrementally. The target range is claimed to be 20 - 60 mg/L (85 - 250 μmol/L).

Felbamate affects the concentrations of a number of other anticonvulsants, increasing concentrations of phenytoin, phenobarbitone and valproate by 25%, but decreasing carbamazepine concentrations by 30% while increasing its epoxide metabolite by 55%. Clearly when felbamate is added to a regimen containing these other anticonvulsants their concentrations need to be checked initially and after every change in its dose. These drugs also decrease felbamate clearance.

Gabapentin

Clinical Use

IMPORTANT FACTS

- Used in partial seizures
- May have a role in bipolar affective disorders

Gabapentin is a lipophilic (aiding blood-brain barrier passage) GABA congener designed to be a GABA agonist. It is useful in partial seizures: simple, complex or partial with secondary generalised tonic-clonic seizures. The mechanism of action is unknown, but may be through release of GABA. Gabapentin has an inter-relationship with calcium-gated channels that is currently unclear. It has similar efficacy to carbamazepine and also, therefore, has a place in the therapy of bipolar disorder. It has also been used in migraine and chronic pain relief. Dosing commences with a low dose with increments to the expected effective therapeutic dose.

Pharmacokinetics

IMPORTANT FACTS
- Gabapentin is not metabolised and is excreted unchanged in urine
- Accumulates in renal failure

Following oral dosing gabapentin is well absorbed, via the L-amino acid transport system. Gabapentin is excreted unchanged, principally in urine with a plasma half-life of 5 - 9 hours. Accumulation can be anticipated in renal failure.

SUMMARY OF GABAPENTIN PHARMACOKINETICS

Parameter	Gabapentin
Oral bioavailability (F)	0.6 - 0.8
Fraction excreted renally	0.65
Fraction bound to plasma proteins	< 0.03
Clearance (corrected for bioavailability) (mL/min/kg)	~ 1.5
Volume of distribution V_d (L/kg)	0.8
Elimination half-life (h)	5 - 7
Time to maximum concentration (h)	2 - 3

Toxicity

Gabapentin has initial moderate side effects that do not normally warrant cessation of dosing, typically comprising fatigue, somnolence, ataxia and dizziness.

Monitoring therapy

IMPORTANT FACT

• Monitoring unnecessary

A target range of 2 - 20 mg/L (12 - 120 µmol/L) has been suggested.

Lamotrigine

Clinical use

IMPORTANT FACTS

• Effective first-line anticonvulsant
• Usable in psychiatric illness
• Phenytoin and phenobarbitone induce metabolism
• Valproate decreases clearance
• Lamotrigine inhibits carbamazepine conversion to epoxide

Lamotrigine was originally introduced as a co-medication with other anticonvulsants for treatment of partial and generalised tonic-clonic seizures, but is now prescribable alone. It was the first of the new anticonvulsants, which are structurally different to the earlier anticonvulsant drugs. It acts by inhibiting the release of excitatory amino acid neurotransmittors. Its profile of action resembles that of carbamazepine and phenytoin including its non-anticonvulsant actions.

Pharmacokinetics

The drug is rapidly and completely absorbed, and maximum plasma concentrations are obtained approximately three hours after oral dosing. The apparent volume of distribution is approximately 1.2 L/kg. Lamotrigine is extensively metabolised in the liver to the glucuronide conjugate, which is then excreted in the urine. Elimination follows linear (first-order) kinetics with a plasma half-life around 24 hours. In the first trimester of pregnancy clearance is increased, it is also significantly affected by concomitant medication with other anticonvulsants. Enzyme-inducing drugs such as phenytoin and carbamazepine reduce the plasma half-life to approximately 15 hours, while treatment with valproic acid prolongs the plasma half-life of lamotrigine to 60 hours. The latter effect may be due to competition between the two drugs for hepatic glucuronidation sites. Lamotrigine may inhibit epoxide hydrolase and delay carbamazepine elimination, precipitating carbamazepine toxicity.

Lamotrigine partitions into breast milk with a ratio of ~ 0.5 - 1.0 milk/plasma.

SUMMARY OF LAMOTRIGINE PHARMACOKINETICS

Parameter	Lamotrigine
Oral bioavailability (F)	~ 1.0
Fraction excreted renally	~ 0.1
Fraction bound to plasma proteins	~ 0.6
Clearance (corrected for bioavailability) (mL/min/kg)	0.4 - 0.6
Volume of distribution V_d (L/kg)	0.9 - 1.2
Elimination half-life (h)	20 - 35
Time to maximum concentration (h)	~ 3

Toxicity

IMPORTANT FACTS

- Combination with other anticonvulsants may be associated with multi-organ failure
- 3 - 5% patients develop rash
- Neurological side effects

Various side effects of lamotrigine therapy have been reported, including rashes (3 - 5% of patients), weakness, visual disturbances, dizziness, drowsiness, unsteadiness, irritability, nausea and gastrointestinal disturbances. Close clinical monitoring (including assessment of hepatic, renal and clotting parameters) is necessary if rash, fever, influenza-like symptoms or worsening of seizure control develop in the early stages of treatment. Lamotrigine in combination with other anticonvulsants has been associated with a rapidly progressive illness with status epilepticus, multi-organ failure and disseminated intravascular coagulation. Lamotrigine's contribution to this syndrome has not been established. There is little evidence of concentration dependent toxicity.

Monitoring therapy

Important fact

- Plasma concentration reflects effect

The variable interactions with other anticonvulsants mentioned above mean that concentration monitoring may be useful in designing a dosing strategy for patients on multiple therapy. A tentative target range of 1 - 4 mg/L (4 - 16 μmol/L) was originally suggested, though this was derived from studies where lamotrigine was used as an adjunct therapy, subsequent studies indicate that values up to 24 mg/L (96 μmol/L) are appropriate in single therapy. However, 5% of subjects suffer side effects at concentrations above 15 mg/L (59 μmol/L), rising to 15% above 20 mg/L (78 μmol/L).

Levetiracetam

Clinical use

Important facts

- Stereoselective
- Adjunct therapy

Levetiracetam is an adjunct therapy in the treatment of partial seizures in adults. Its mechanism of action is unknown; it does not act on sodium gated channels, or on GABA or glutamate receptors. The fact that it is the S-enantiomer of the pyrrolidine α–ethyl-2-oxo-1-pyrrolidineacetamide indicates a stereoselective binding site.

Pharmacokinetics

Important facts

- Predominantly excreted unchanged
- Accumulates in renal failure
- No significant drug-drug interactions

Following virtually complete absorption levetiracetam is mainly excreted as unchanged drug, ~ 65%, with a further ~ 25% excreted following hydrolysis of the acetamide group. As it is not metabolised by cytochrome enzymes it does not have any significant interactions with drugs metabolised by these enzymes i.e. other anticonvulsants, anticoagulants or oral contraceptives. Its renal excretion means that the plasma half-life is longer in the elderly. Dose reduction is necessary at creatinine clearances below 60 mL/min/1.73 m^2.

SUMMARY OF LEVETIRACETAM PHARMACOKINETICS

Parameter	Levetiracetam
Oral bioavailability (F)	~ 1.0
Fraction excreted renally	~ 0.7
Fraction bound to plasma proteins	< 0.1
Clearance (corrected for bioavailability) (mL/min/kg)	~ 1.0
Volume of distribution V_d (L/kg)	0.5 - 0.7
Elimination half-life (h)	6 - 8
Time to maximum concentration (h)	0.5 - 1.0

Toxicity

IMPORTANT FACT

- Levetiracetam has a good safety profile

Levetiracetam has a very good safety profile, increasing doses being generally well tolerated. The principal adverse effects listed in increasing frequency are asthenia, dizziness and somnolence.

Monitoring therapy

- There is no evidence to justify monitoring levetiracetam other than to assess adherence, though a range of 6 - 20 mg/L (35 - 118 μmol/L) has been suggested.

Oxcarbazepine

Clinical use

IMPORTANT FACTS

- Carbamazepine analogue
- 10-hydroxy metabolite active
- Less between subject variability in pharmacokinetics than carbamazepine

Oxcarbazepine is the 10-keto analogue of carbamazepine and has been used in Europe from the early 1990s, and more recently in the US, for the treatment of general tonic-clonic or partial onset seizures. Oxcarbazepine has an active metabolite, 10-hydroxycarbazepine; both exert their effect in a manner similar to carbamazepine through stabilisation of hyperexcited neural membranes and inhibition of repetitive neuronal firing. The advantage of oxcarbazepine over carbamazepine is that the former has less variable kinetics.

Pharmacokinetics

IMPORTANT FACTS

- First-pass non-cytochrome metabolism
- Non-inducible metabolism
- Reductive metabolism
- Pro-drug for monohydroxycarbazepine

Unlike carbamazepine, oxcarbazepine is not extensively metabolised by the cytochrome enzyme system, but is metabolised to the 10-hydroxy metabolite by cytosolic arylketone reductase; this is a first-pass effect and is rapid. Phase one metabolism proceeds to the formation of carbazepine 10,11-trans-dihydrodiol and phase two to glucuronidation of the monohydroxy metabolite (~ 70%).

In contrast to carbamazepine the metabolism of oxcarbazepine is not inducible (unusually) nor is it oxidative. The reductive metabolism is rapid and high capacity resulting in very little oxcarbazine, making oxcarbazepine effectively a pro-drug for monohydroxyoxcarbazepine.

Doses of oxcarbazepine are up to 1200 mg/day with complete absorption. Oxcarbazepine half-life is under 2 hours. Monohydroxycarbazepine has a half-life of between 8-12 hours, a volume of distribution of 49 litres in a 70 kg man and a time to peak concentration of around 4.5 hours.

SUMMARY OF OXCARBAZEPINE PHARMACOKINETICS
(O = OXCARBAZEPINE, H = HYDROXY METABOLITE)

Parameter	O	H
Oral bioavailability (F)	1.0	NA
Fraction excreted renally	< 0.01	~ 0.3
Fraction bound to plasma proteins	0.6	~ 0.5
Clearance (corrected for bioavailability) (mL/min/kg)	~ 0.7	NA
Volume of distribution V_d (L/kg)	4	0.7
Elimination half-life (h)	~ 2	8 - 16
Time to maximum concentration (h) (im/iv)	1 - 3	2 - 6

Toxicity

IMPORTANT FACTS

- Less liver damage than carbamazepine
- High incidence of hyponatraemia
- Similar neurological side effects to carbamazepine

Oxcarbazepine is not subject to the range of interactions or liver damage experienced with carbamazepine. However, that is not to say that oxcarbazepine does not have side effects. There is a high incidence, ~ 25%, of hyponatraemia (< 125 mmol/L), presumably related to an inappropriate antidiuresis, which resolves on cessation of treatment. Neurological side effects mimic those of carbamazepine.

Monitoring therapy

IMPORTANT FACT

- Monitoring unnecessary

There is little published evidence validating the need to measure oxcarbazepine and/or its metabolite, consequently there are no commercially available immunoassays. Measurements are typically done by HPLC. A range of 13 - 28 µg/L (50 - 110 µmol/L) has been suggested. Drugs metabolised via the CYP2C19 and CYP3A4/5 isoenzymes will be inhibited by oxcarbazepine, though to a lesser extent than is the case for carbamazepine. The AUCs of the oral contraceptives ethinylestradiol and levonorgestrel were reduced by ~ 50% by oxcarbazepine, concomitant use is contraindicated.

Phenobarbital (and Primidone)

Clinical use

IMPORTANT FACTS

- Previously widely used, now minor anticonvulsants
- Primidone is a pro-drug, never used now

Phenobarbital, first introduced in 1912, was the first effective organic antiepileptic agent, but is now of minority interest. Phenobarbital monotherapy has been shown to be inferior to monotherapy with carbamazepine or phenytoin in producing complete control of seizures when used as initial treatment, and the sedative effects (in adults) and behavioural disturbances (in children) are trouble-some. It is a third-line drug for tonic or partial seizures, and is also used for the prophylaxis of febrile convulsions in children at particularly high risk. Phenobarbital is not indicated for absence seizures. In common with other anti-convulsants, it limits the spread of seizure activity and raises the seizure threshold. At therapeutic concentrations, phenobarbital can reduce the excitatory effects of glutamate and augment the inhibitory effects of gamma-aminobutyric acid (GABA). Phenobarbital is now rarely used in Europe, but still finds favour in the US.

Pharmacokinetics

IMPORTANT FACTS

- Very long plasma half-life
- Induces its own metabolism

Oral absorption of phenobarbital is complete but slow, and peak concentrations do not occur until several hours after a single dose. Approximately 40 - 60% of the drug is protein-bound in plasma, and the volume of distribution approximates to total body water, around 0.6 L/kg. Up to 30% of an oral dose is eliminated unchanged in the urine, and excretion is pH dependent. The remaining drug is inactivated by microsomal oxidation. The plasma half-life is long, typically 100 hours in adults, which means that three weeks or more may be required to reach steady-state concentrations after initiation or alteration of therapy. The plasma half-life is longer in neonates, and shorter and more variable in children.

SUMMARY OF PHENOBARBITAL PHARMACOKINETICS

Parameter	Phenobarbital
Oral bioavailability (F)	~ 1.0
Fraction excreted renally	~ 0.25
Fraction bound to plasma proteins	~ 0.5
Clearance (corrected for bioavailability) (mL/min/kg)	0.05 - 0.08
Volume of distribution V_d (L/kg)	~ 0.6
Elimination half-life (h)	80 - 120
Time to maximum concentration (h)	2 - 4

Toxicity

IMPORTANT FACTS

- Sedative
- 1 - 2% have rash
- Nystagmus and ataxia

The most frequent undesirable effect of phenobarbital is sedation, which occurs in most patients on starting treatment. However, tolerance develops on chronic medication. Other signs of excessive dosage include nystagmus and ataxia. Paradoxical excitement, restlessness and confusion may occur in the elderly, and hyperkinesia in children. A rash appears in 1 to 2% of patients. Megaloblastic anaemia responding to folate, and osteomalacia responding to high dose vitamin D, may also occur as a consequence of the drug's ability to induce hepatic enzyme systems. The babies of mothers taking phenobarbital during pregnancy sometimes develop hypoprothrombinaemia with haemorrhage soon after birth. Vitamin K is effective for treatment or prophylaxis.

Monitoring therapy

IMPORTANT FACTS

- Target range should be interpreted flexibly
- Tolerance develops
- Valproate causes plasma concentrations to rise significantly
- Poor correlation between plasma concentration and effect

Tolerance to the pharmacological effects of phenobarbital develops on long-term therapy, a fact which complicates the interpretation of plasma drug concentrations. A target range of 10 - 40 mg/L (40 - 160 µmol/L) is frequently said to be associated with optimal control, but these limits must be interpreted with considerable flexibility. In particular, very low concentrations of phenobarbital, well below the lower limit of the target range, may have a significant antiepileptic effect in patients who have been on the drug for a long time, and withdrawal of the drug under these circumstances may provoke marked rebound seizures.

The development of tolerance also means that there is poor correlation between plasma concentrations and adverse effects. Naive patients may exhibit marked drowsiness at concentrations as low as 5 mg/L (20 µmol/L), while others on long-term therapy may tolerate concentrations up to 60 mg/L (260 µmol/L) with no apparent ill effects. Phenobarbital concentrations of 15 - 20 mg/L (65 - 85 µmol/L) are generally accepted as providing effective prophylaxis against febrile convulsion in children.

If valproate is added to an existing phenobarbital regime, plasma phenobarbital concentrations increase sharply in the majority of patients, and a reduction in dosage is usually required. Concentration monitoring may be useful in this situation.

The pKa of phenobarbital is 7.3, and the concentration in saliva is therefore highly dependent upon changes in salivary pH, which in turn depends on flow rate. This means that salivary monitoring is not suitable for routine monitoring of therapy.

The poor correlation between plasma drug concentrations and clinical and toxic effects means that one of the cardinal requirements of therapeutic drug monitoring is not fulfilled for phenobarbital. Routine monitoring is thus of very limited value, although plasma concentration data may occasionally be useful in improving compliance, minimising the effects of drug interactions or confirming a clinical diagnosis of intoxication, provided the limitations of the measurement are understood. Monitoring is also valuable in children receiving the drug for prophylaxis of febrile convulsions, to ensure that adequate concentrations have been achieved. The long half-life of phenobarbital means that timing of samples in relationship to dosage is generally unimportant. Primidone monitoring is through plasma phenobarbital measurement.

Phenytoin

Clinical use

IMPORTANT FACTS

- Still widely used, usually with other anticonvulsants
- Poor side effect profile
- Saturation kinetics
- Long plasma half-life
- No longer first choice in status epilepticus
- Used for trigeminal neuralgia

Phenytoin was introduced in 1938 having been discovered as a result of an animal model screening process; it remains a widely used primary anticonvulsant drug for the prophylaxis and treatment of generalised tonic-clonic, grand mal, focal and partial seizures. With the aid of careful plasma concentration monitoring, it has been claimed around 80% of newly diagnosed epileptic patients can be controlled on phenytoin alone, however the side effect profile means it is no longer a first choice drug.

Like carbamazepine, the drug acts by inhibition of voltage-gated sodium channels and is thought to reduce the spread of excitation from epileptic foci. Phenytoin has a relatively long plasma half-life, and is particularly useful when once daily dosing is appropriate, such as in alcohol related epilepsy or in the elderly. It is less suitable for use in young female patients because of the unpleasant cosmetic effects that may develop (coarse facies, acne, hirsutism and gingival hyperplasia), and carbamazepine or sodium valproate may be preferred initially for such patients.

Intravenous phenytoin is effective in the management of status epilepticus, but benzodiazepines are safer and are used more frequently. Other applications include the management of trigeminal neuralgia if carbamazepine has proved ineffective or intolerable.

Pharmacokinetics

IMPORTANT FACTS

- Variable, occasionally incomplete, absorption
- Metabolised by the cytochrome P450 isoenzyme CYP2C9
- Zero-order kinetics, small increases in dose cause large increases in plasma concentration
- Consequently half-life not readily predictable

Absorption of phenytoin given orally is slow, sometimes variable and occasionally incomplete, although bioavailability is normally around 90%. The primary determinant of absorption is particle size, which is affected by the dosage form and the excipients used. Marked changes in concentration profile have occurred in the past on changing formulation.

Phenytoin is approximately 90% bound to plasma proteins, principally albumin, in healthy adults taking the drug as monotherapy. Protein binding is substantially lower in a number of situations, notably patients with renal or hepatic disease, neonates, and in the last trimester of pregnancy. Concurrent therapy with sodium valproate displaces phenytoin from protein binding sites, reducing the total plasma phenytoin concentration while increasing the free fraction.

Phenytoin is metabolised by oxidation by CYP2C9 in the liver. The most important feature of its pharmacokinetics is the limited capacity of the hepatic mixed-function oxidase system, which can become saturated at plasma phenytoin concentrations within the target range. Consequently the drug exhibits dose-dependent pharmacokinetics. As the plasma concentration rises the metabolic capacity is exceeded and clearance (and hence elimination half-life) falls with clinically important sequelae. Initially, prior to saturation, the kinetics are linear, beyond saturation they are non-linear, the result is a small increase in dose or a small change in metabolic capacity (e.g. due to intercurrent illness) can result in large increases in plasma concentration and precipitate toxicity. The plasma concentration at which saturation is approached varies between individual patients and this contributes to the large inter-individual differences in plasma phenytoin concentrations in patients on the same dose of the drug (see Figure 1.1).

The phenomenon of saturation kinetics also means that plasma half-lives get longer as plasma concentrations increase, and thus the range of observed half-lives is wide although, strictly speaking, half-life is not a valid concept for a drug which exhibits saturation kinetics. Premature babies have very long elimination half-lives (due to immaturity of the hepatic mixed function oxidase system), which shorten markedly to around half that found in adults, in infancy and childhood.

The main metabolite of phenytoin produced in the liver is para-hydroxyphenyl phenylhydantoin (HPPH), which is inactive. This metabolite is conjugated with glucuronic acid and excreted in the urine. A number of minor phase one metabolites are also formed, which go on to be conjugated with glucuronic acid. Patients with renal failure may accumulate high levels of HPPH in the plasma, which may cross-react in some immunoassays and give misleading results.

SUMMARY OF PHENYTOIN PHARMACOKINETICS

Parameter	Phenytoin
Oral bioavailability (F)	0.9
Fraction excreted renally	< 0.1
Fraction bound to plasma proteins	0.9
Clearance (corrected for bioavailability) (mL/min/kg)	Varies with concentration
Volume of distribution V_d (L/kg)	0.65
Elimination half-life (h)	6 - 24
Time to maximum concentration (h)	3 - 12

Toxicity

IMPORTANT FACTS

- Neurotoxicity
- Chronic side effects may be disabling or disfiguring
- Idiosyncratic toxic reactions
- Paradoxical seizures

Phenytoin has a low therapeutic index and exhibits a number of troublesome concentration dependent side effects. Symptoms of neurotoxicity (nystagmus, nausea, vomiting, drowsiness, dysarthria, tremor and ataxia) become increasingly apparent as plasma concentrations exceed 20 mg/L (80 μmol/L). High plasma phenytoin concentrations may increase the frequency of fits (so-called paradoxical seizures). These are clinically indistinguishable from epileptiform seizures and are an indication for urgent plasma concentration measurement to aid discrimination of the cause in a patient presenting to the Accident and Emergency Department. Prolonged toxic phenytoin concentrations have been associated with irreversible peripheral nerve or cerebellar damage. Intellectual deterioration, depression, behavioural problems, reduced drive and initiative, and psychomotor slowing are more subtle long-term problems associated with phenytoin.

Idiosyncratic effects include the cosmetic effects mentioned above, plus erythroderma, hepatotoxicity, blood dyscrasias and systemic lupus erythematosus. Long-term phenytoin use may be associated with osteomalacia and folate-dependent megaloblastic anaemia. Developmental abnormalities occur in about 10% of the offspring of women taking phenytoin during the early stages of pregnancy.

Monitoring therapy

IMPORTANT FACTS

- Target range 5 - 20 mg/L (20 - 80 μmol/L)
- Treat the patient not the concentration
- There is no correlation of effect with dose
- Plasma concentrations correlate well with effect
- Saliva concentrations reflect plasma concentrations
- Free phenytoin plasma concentrations correlate best with effect
- Dose changes should be judicious
- Monitor iv regimens when used for status epilepticus
- Clearance increased in pregnancy
- Drug interactions require consideration

Early studies clearly demonstrated improved control of generalised tonic-clonic and partial seizures with plasma phenytoin concentrations greater than 10 mg/L (40 μmol/L). As clinical signs of toxicity become apparent in many patients above 20 mg/L (80 μmol/L), the original lower limit of the target range of 10 mg/L (40 μmol/L) has been modified to 5 mg/L (20 μmol/L) and some patients respond below this concentration. Conversely, seizure control may only be complete in some patients with plasma concentrations substantially greater than 20 mg/L (80 μmol/L). In the absence of unacceptable toxicity, misguided attempts to reduce the plasma phenytoin concentration in such patients are likely to precipitate the loss of seizure control. Clinical judgement is paramount in interpreting results. The case for routine concentration monitoring of phenytoin is stronger than for most other therapeutic agents.

Measurement of phenytoin in saliva is feasible and valid, but has a number of practical disadvantages and is not widely practised for routine monitoring.

However, despite studies demonstrating that free phenytoin concentrations correlate best with the clinical situation and despite being relatively easy to measure, free concentrations are rarely monitored in the UK; this is in marked contrast to US and European practice. The target range is 10% of the total range i.e. 0.5 - 2 mg/L (2 - 8 μmol/L). Changes in binding due to changes in albumin concentrations or displacement caused by metabolic changes induced by disease e.g. renal failure or displacement by other drugs are all indications for free drug concentration monitoring.

The main indications for monitoring are as follows:

On initiating therapy. The dose should be tailored to produce concentrations likely to be clinically effective without producing toxicity. Phenytoin is used prophylactically following neurosurgery and dose optimisation cannot rely on previous results; frequent monitoring is advisable. It may well be that pre-operative determination of CYP2C9, the predominant cytochrome enzyme responsible for phenytoin metabolism may allow optimal dosing in this circumstance.

When seizures are infrequent, measuring the plasma concentration can give some idea of the likelihood of control. Concentration monitoring can also guide dosage increases if seizure control is inadequate. If the plasma concentration is below 5 mg/L (20 μmol/L), an increment in daily dose of 100 mg is usually appropriate. Between 5 and 15 mg/L (20 - 60 μmol/L), the dose increase should not exceed 50 mg/day, and at plasma concentrations above 15 mg/L (60 μmol/L) dose increments should be only 25 mg/day because of the high risk of saturation of metabolism and large increases in plasma concentration.

During intravenous therapy in status epilepticus. The long half-life means that the phenytoin concentration may remain within the target range for up to 24 hours after a bolus dose. Concentration monitoring at intervals after a loading dose aids the choice and timing of maintenance therapy.

Unexpected deterioration in seizure control. When a regime previously shown to give good seizure control suddenly fails to control fits, concentration monitoring may identify poor adherence, altered pharmacokinetics e.g. bioavailability, or a reduction in seizure threshold due to some intercurrent problem.

As an adjunct to the diagnosis of toxicity. As indicated above, some patients tolerate phenytoin concentrations above the target range much better than others, and acute toxic concentrations may be necessary in these cases for optimal control. It is always necessary to question and examine the patient to ascertain if toxicity is present. However, in a patient with signs and symptoms of phenytoin toxicity, concentration measurement may confirm the diagnosis and guide the degree of dosage reduction. The impact of chronic toxicity in such patients should be borne in mind.

When interacting drugs are added or withdrawn. A wide variety of drugs alter phenytoin metabolism, usually by induction or inhibition of the enzyme systems involved. Reduced absorption and displacement of phenytoin from binding proteins are also seen with some drugs. It seems prudent to monitor phenytoin concentrations when such drugs are introduced or withdrawn.

In pregnancy. Phenytoin clearance is accelerated in pregnancy, and seizure control may be adversely affected. If phenytoin therapy must be continued during pregnancy (the risks of stopping the drug frequently outweigh the risks of continuing), monthly monitoring is advisable and the aim is to maintain the minimum effective dose. Small falls in concentration may reflect decreased protein binding, and do not warrant increasing the dose if the patient remains free of convulsions, free phenytoin concentration measurement is warranted if there is clinical doubt. Deteriorating seizure control or large falls in phenytoin concentration obviously require a dose increase.

Tiagabine

Clinical use

IMPORTANT FACT

- Adjunct therapy

Tiagabine is a nipecotic acid inhibitor of GAT-1, the GABA transporter. It acts by inhibiting GABA uptake, thereby prolonging its effect at inhibitory synapses. As adjunct therapy it is useful against partial seizures.

Pharmacokinetics

IMPORTANT FACTS

- Metabolised by the cytochrome P450 isoenzyme CYP3A
- Hepatic enzyme-inducing anticonvulsants increase clearance

Tiagabine is well absorbed on oral administration and while it is highly bound to plasma proteins it is mainly metabolised by hepatic CYP3A with a half-life of around 8 hours. However, co-administration with enzyme-inducing anticonvulsants decreases the plasma half-life to ~ 3 hours.

SUMMARY OF TIAGABINE PHARMACOKINETICS

Parameter	Tiagabine
Oral bioavailability (F)	~ 0.9
Fraction excreted renally	< 0.05
Fraction bound to plasma proteins	~ 0.95
Clearance (corrected for bioavailability) (mL/min/kg)	1.5 - 2.5
Volume of distribution V_d (L/kg)	0.9 - 1.7
Elimination half-life (h)	7 - 9
Time to maximum concentration (h)	0.5 - 2.5

Toxicity

Mild side effects of tremor, dizziness and somnolence pass soon after commencement of therapy.

Monitoring therapy

IMPORTANT FACTS

- No strong evidence for monitoring
- There is a lack of correlation between plasma concentration and effect, 20 - 40 µg/L may be a target range.

Topiramate

Clinical use

IMPORTANT FACTS

- Adjunct therapy
- Monotherapy may be effective

Usable as an adjunct therapy, topiramate inhibits voltage gated sodium channels, possibly by a mechanism similar to phenytoin. Topiramate has other mechanisms of action too, inhibiting one form of glutamate receptor and influencing post-synaptic GABA flux. Structurally topiramate is a monosaccharide with a sulfamate substitution, it has a wide spectrum of activity being effective in tonic-clonic seizures, refractory partial seizures, Lennox-Gastaut syndrome, drop attacks and possibly infantile spasm. Some work has been done on the use of topiramate as monotherapy, which would appear to be successful.

Pharmacokinetics

Oral absorption is rapid with ~ 90% being excreted unchanged in urine, the phase one and two metabolites account for the remainder and have no pharmacological activity; the plasma half-life is ~ 24 hours. Clearance increases if carbamazepine is given simultaneously and felbamate has an even greater effect.

SUMMARY OF TOPIRAMATE PHARMACOKINETICS

Parameter	Topiramate
Oral bioavailability (F)	~ 0.8
Fraction excreted renally	~ 0.9
Fraction bound to plasma proteins	~ 0.15
Clearance (corrected for bioavailability) (mL/min/kg)	0.3 - 0.5
Volume of distribution V_d (L/kg)	0.6 - 0.8
Elimination half-life (h)	20 - 30
Time to maximum concentration (h)	1 - 2.5

Toxicity

Topiramate is generally well tolerated. While side effects are mild below a plasma concentration of 25 mg/L (75 μmol/L), they are significantly worse above this concentration.

Monitoring therapy

Plasma concentrations below 25 mg/L (75 μmol/L) are said to be well tolerated.

Valproic Acid

Clinical use

IMPORTANT FACTS

- A first-line anticonvulsant
- Good side effect profile
- Usable in bipolar affective disorder

Valproic acid has a different spectrum of anticonvulsant activity from the above anticonvulsants, and it is the drug of choice for the treatment of myoclonic seizures and generalised absence seizures, where its minimal sedative action and absence of CNS side effects make it a first-line drug (along with phenytoin and carbamazepine). It is also effective in general and partial epilepsy. Valproate has also been used in the prophylaxis of febrile convulsions, though whether it is the drug of choice is controversial. Valproate is believed to act through GABA accumulation and enhancing post-synaptic GABA response.

Valproate is an effective option in the therapy of bipolar affective disorder.

Pharmacokinetics

Valproic acid has a complex pharmacokinetic profile. It is strongly bound to plasma proteins, and this binding is concentration dependent so that the free fraction (and hence the apparent clearance) rises with plasma concentration being ~ 90 % bound up to around 80 mg/L (320 μmol/L) and decreasing thereafter. At high doses of valproate, therefore, further dose increases may result in a smaller than expected rise in circulating concentration. Plasma protein binding is reduced, and clearance enhanced, in pregnancy and in patients with renal failure. Free fatty acids in plasma displace valproate from binding sites on albumin, and clearance of the drug is different in the fasting and fed states. This helps to explain the wide circadian variation in valproate pharmacokinetics, and the observation that plasma concentrations may vary by as much as 100% across the dosage interval. Even consecutive fasting concentrations in patients on twice-daily dosing are not reproducible. Valproate clearance is also increased by other anticonvulsants, notably phenytoin and phenobarbitone.

The volume of distribution of valproic acid is small, ~ 0.1 - 0.5 L/kg and the drug is primarily cleared (> 95 %) from plasma by hepatic metabolism by a variety of mechanisms including: β-oxidation, ω-hydroxylation and glucuronidation; the principal metabolite is 4-en-valproic acid (thought to be responsible for hepatotoxicity). The metabolite 2-N-propyl-3-oxo-pentanoic acid, has similar activity to valproic acid. The plasma half-life of the unchanged drug is relatively short (6 - 16 hours), but the major metabolites have much slower elimination rates. This helps to explain the observation that the maximal anticonvulsant effect of valproic acid is usually not observed during the initial phase of treatment, even though steady state concentrations have been achieved. Further, seizure control and control of bipolar affective disorder frequently persist after the drug has been stopped and intact drug has been cleared from the circulation.

SUMMARY OF VALPROATE PHARMACOKINETICS

Parameter	Valproate
Oral bioavailability (F)	~ 1.0
Fraction excreted renally	< 0.05
Fraction bound to plasma proteins	~ 0.95
Clearance (corrected for bioavailability) (mL/min/kg)	~ 0.1
Volume of distribution V_d (L/kg)	0.15 - 0.3
Elimination half-life (h)	11 - 17
Time to maximum concentration (h)	1 - 4

Toxicity

IMPORTANT FACTS

- Weight gain occurs
- Rare dermatological and haematological reactions
- Paediatric patients at risk of hepatotoxicity
- Hyperammonaemia can occur
- Teratogenic

The most common side effect of valproate therapy is weight gain, followed by nausea, tremor and vomiting; the latter symptoms occur less frequently with enteric coated tablets, reducing the incidence to below 5%. Alopecia, skin rashes and haematological reactions (thrombocytopenia and inhibition of platelet aggregation) occur rarely.

A rare but serious complication of valproate therapy is the development of serious hepatotoxicity in children under 2 years with an overall mortality rate estimated at about 1 in 5000. This is related to the high free radical load generated by valproate therapy and the inability of the susceptible individuals' glutathione peroxidase to cope. Multiple anticonvulsant therapy is said to increase the risk of death. The onset is usually during the first six months of therapy. Vomiting, lethargy and drowsiness precede the development of jaundice and are a clear indication for immediate cessation of therapy. Increasing seizure frequency, hepatic coma and death may develop. Biochemical testing is unhelpful in predicting liver damage as many patients show transient elevations of transaminases during the early months of therapy.

Various metabolic derangements have been associated with valproate treatment, and the drug inhibits urea synthesis and causes hyperammonaemia. Ideally, urea cycle defects should be excluded before starting an infant on the drug.

There is an association between valproate therapy in pregnancy and open spina bifida, and if the drug is continued during pregnancy ultrasound scanning and early amniocentesis should be offered.

Monitoring therapy

IMPORTANT FACTS

- Pharmacokinetic studies indicate a poor relationship with pharmaco-dynamics
- Most authorities agree routine monitoring is not necessary
- Psychiatric applications find monitoring useful when compliance is an issue

Hard evidence for a target range of valproate concentrations does not exist. Studies indicate that plasma concentrations are no better a guide to clinical response than is the dose, and definitive data to support the original tentative range of 50 - 100 mg/L (350 - 700 μmol/L) are not available, despite the frequency with which this range is quoted. It is clear that some patients are effectively controlled with concentrations below 50 mg/L (350 μmol/L) and others require concentrations far in excess of 100 mg/L (700 μmol/L). Toxic effects also show no clear relationship to plasma concentration, this plus the large inter-dose variations in kinetics noted above, are the reasons that monitoring valproate concentrations is not helpful.

Most authorities now agree that routine monitoring of valproate concentrations should not be practised. It is unnecessary and potentially misleading, since it is not possible to relate a single concentration measurement to the clinical effect in any meaningful fashion. Free (unbound) or salivary concentrations are no more useful in relation to seizure control. There is a crude correlation with the likelihood of CNS toxicity when concentrations exceed 100 mg/L (700 μmol/L), although many patients tolerate much higher concentrations without complaint and with benefit.

Measurement may be useful in the event of therapeutic failure in spite of apparently adequate dosing. In this setting, a concentration consistently above approximately 140 mg/L (1000 μmol/L) suggests that an alternative anticonvulsant should be substituted. However, despite the kinetics being the same, a similar range of 50 - 125 mg/L (350 - 870 μmol/L) is adhered to in psychiatry with greater rigour. Monitoring is performed to document tolerance to treatment on initiation of therapy, with less frequent monitoring once therapy is established.

Vigabatrin

Clinical use

IMPORTANT FACT

- Increasing use as mono- and adjunct therapy

Vigabatrin is a now widely licensed in Europe for use in chronic epilepsy not controlled satisfactorily by other anticonvulsants. It is a structural analogue of the inhibitory neurotransmitter γ-aminobutyric acid (GABA), and was designed specifically as an anticonvulsant. The drug acts as a specific irreversible inhibitor of GABA transferase, the enzyme responsible for GABA catabolism.

Pharmacokinetics
Vigabatrin is rapidly absorbed following oral administration, with peak plasma concentrations occuring between 0.7 and 2 hours post-dose. The lack of an intravenous preparation makes absolute bioavailability difficult to determine, but most of an oral dose is absorbed.

The drug is chiral, and is supplied as a racemic R/S mixture. The R(-) isomer is inactive, and only the S(+) isomer possesses pharmacological activity. The pharmacokinetic properties of the active S(+) isomer appear generally similar to those of the racemate, but it remains important to use stereoselective assays in pharmacokinetic studies to avoid the production of misleading data. For example, studies on the overall clearance of (R,S)-vigabatrin in children indicate that clearance increases with age, suggesting that older children will need higher doses of the drug. However, stereoselective methods show that clearance only increases with age for the R(-) inactive isomer. Clearance of the active isomer is independent of age and there is no reason for age-related dosing. Distribution studies suggest that the volume of distribution for the S(+) isomer is slightly larger than for the R(-) isomer.

Vigabatrin is minimally metabolised, and the major route of elimination is by renal excretion of the unchanged drug. Surprisingly, vigabatrin has been reported to produce a fall of about 20% in circulating phenytoin concentrations when used in patients already receiving phenytoin. Other anticonvulsants are unaffected and the mechanism of the effect is not clear.

SUMMARY OF VIGABATRIN PHARMACOKINETICS

Parameter	Vigabatrin
Oral bioavailability (F)	0.8
Fraction excreted renally	0.7
Fraction bound to plasma proteins	0
Clearance (corrected for bioavailability) (mL/min/kg)	1.3
Volume of distribution V_d (L/kg)	0.8
Elimination half-life (h)	6 - 8
Time to maximum concentration (h)	0.5 - 2.0

Toxicity

IMPORTANT FACTS

- Generally good side effect profile
- Some serious side effects

Few adverse effects have been described. The most common side effect is a dose-related drowsiness, dizziness and ataxia. Prominent behavioural side effects (aggression and psychosis) are a problem in some patients. More worryingly there have been reports of irreversible visual field defects. Hyperactivity and agitation are the most frequent side effects in children.

Monitoring therapy

- Monitoring unnecessary

Vigabatrin plasma concentrations are related to dosage, but there is no clear corre-lation between plasma concentration and clinical effect. This is related to the mechanism of action of the drug. Although the circulating half-life is short, viga-batrin's duration of action exceeds 24 h as a consequence of its irreversible binding to the target enzyme in the brain. In clinical studies, the full effects of increasing and decreasing vigabatrin dosage did not become apparent until 2 - 10 days after the change.

Routine monitoring of plasma concentrations is unnecessary. If monitoring is required, for example in specialised pharmacokinetic or toxicological studies, stereoselective methods capable of differentiating between the R(-) and S(+) enan-tiomers are required.

Zonisamide

Clinical use

- Adjunct therapy

Zonisamide is structurally related to the sulfonamides and is an adjunct therapy for partial seizures. Introduced recently, its efficacy against other seizures remains to be established. It is a broad spectrum anticonvulsant blocking both sodium and calcium gated channels; it also inhibits carbonic anhydrase.

Pharmacokinetics
Following oral administration zonisamide is almost completely absorbed and ~ 30% is excreted unchanged in the urine. The remainder is metabolised to sulfamoylacetylphenol glucuronide via CYP3A4, consequently concomitant administration with drugs such as phenytoin, carbamazepine and phenobarbi-tone cause an approximate 50% decrease in the uninduced plasma half-life of ~ 65 hours; conversely lamotrigine appears to inhibit clearance, however there are conflicting reports. The unchanged drug is ~ 40% bound to plasma proteins. Zonisamide is significantly bound to red cell components, this is saturable and is

maximised before the therapeutically effective concentrations of 10 - 20 µg/L (47 - 94 µmol/L) are reached and therefore is not a consideration in therapy.

Summary of zonisamide pharmacokinetics

Parameter	Zonisamide
Oral bioavailability (F)	~ 1.0
Fraction excreted renally	~ 0.3
Fraction bound to plasma proteins	~ 0.4
Clearance (corrected for bioavailability) (mL/min/kg)	0.5
Volume of distribution V_d (L/kg)	~ 1.0
Elimination half-life (h)	~ 65
Time to maximum concentration (h)	2.0

Toxicity

Zonisamide is generally well tolerated, though mild side effects such as tiredness and ataxia can occur. There is reported to be a 1% incidence of renal calculi, the cause of which is unknown.

Monitoring therapy

Important fact

 • Monitoring may be relevant

Concentrations of 10 - 20 mg/L (47 - 94 µmol/L) are achieved in therapy and are well tolerated, with toxicity occurring above 40 mg/L (190 µmol/L). The interaction with other anticonvulsants allows that the concept of monitoring zonisamide might have relevance.

Structures of some anticonvulsants

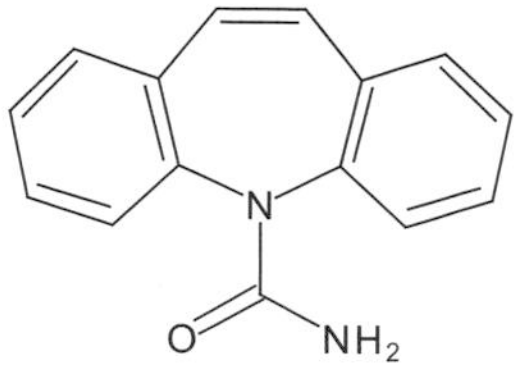

Carbamazepine

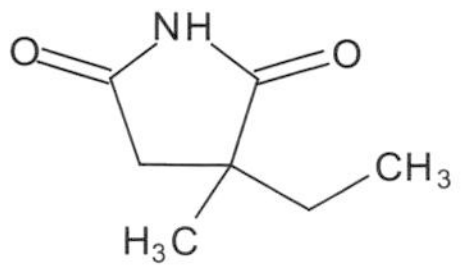

Ethosuximide

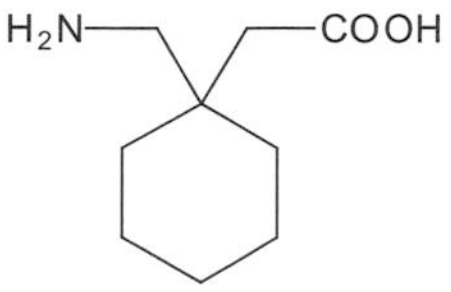

Gabapentin

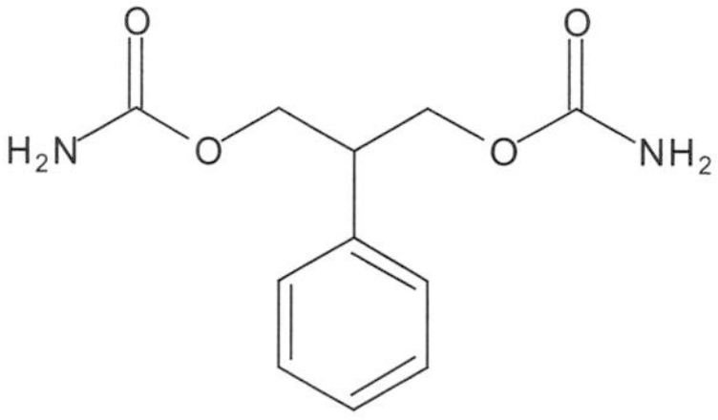

Felbamate

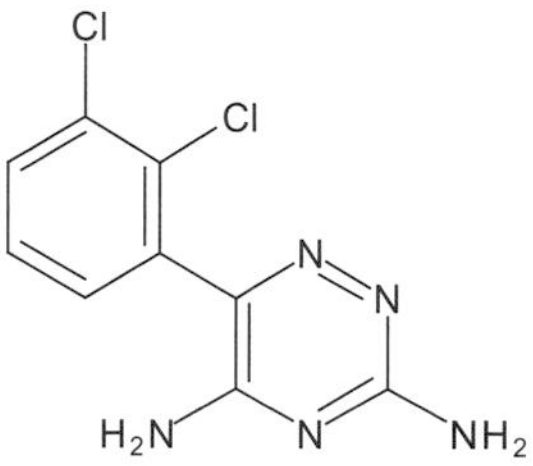

Lamotrigine

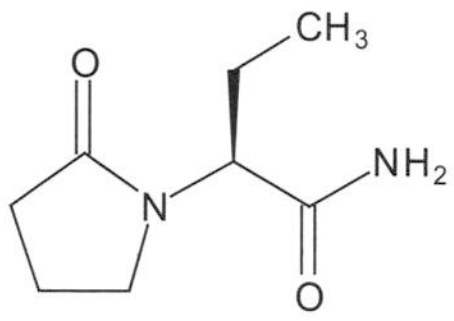

Levetiracetam

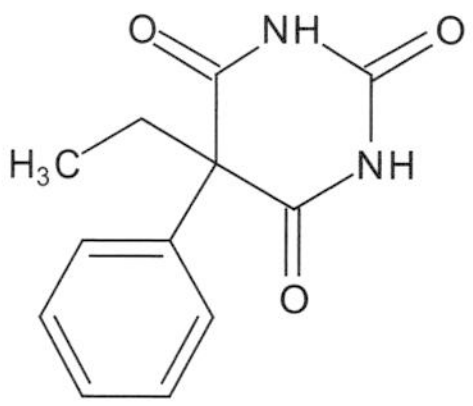

Phenobarbital

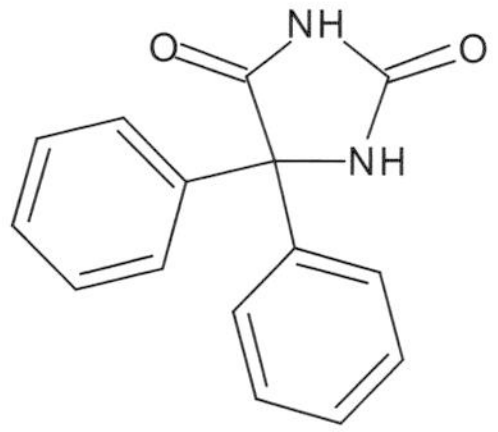

Phenytoin

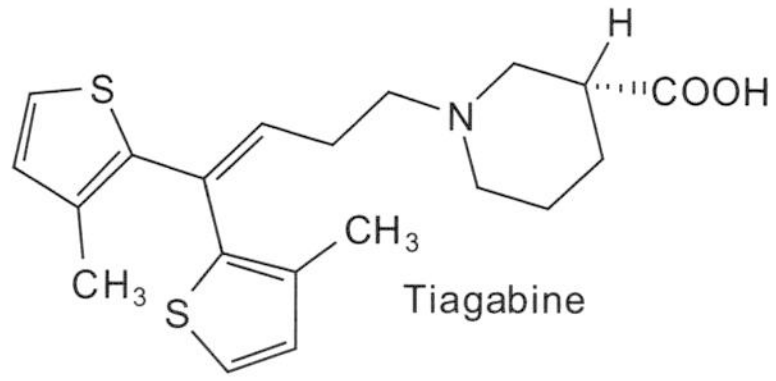

Tiagabine

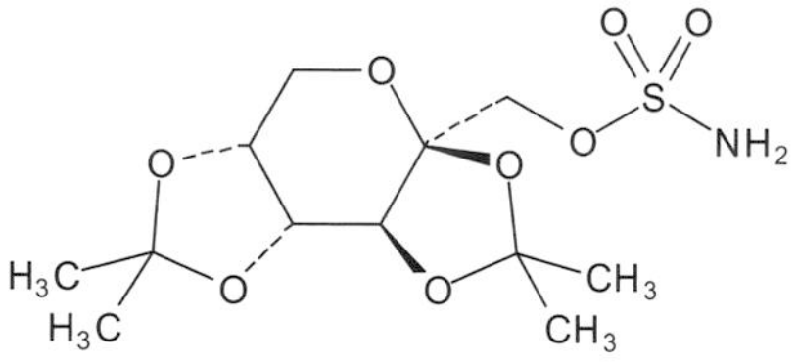

Topiramate

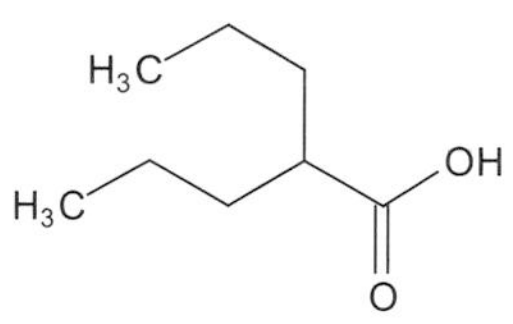

Valproic acid

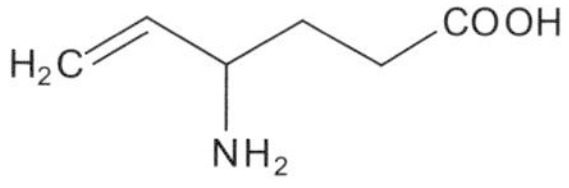

Vigabatrin

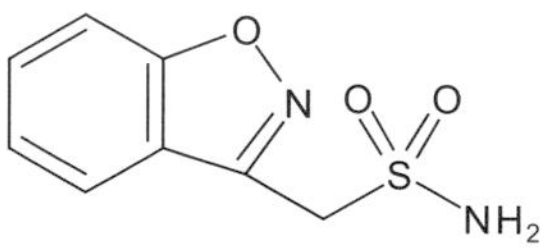

Zonisamide

ANTIDEPRESSANTS

General

Since the first edition of this book, treatment with antidepressants has undergone a revolution. Tricyclic antidepressants (TCAs) had been the mainstay of drug therapy for many years. The need for TDM was well described, albeit practiced more widely outside the UK. While there is a relationship between efficacy, toxicity and plasma concentration, TCA therapy was associated with significant anticholinergic side effects. TCAs are dangerous in overdose with a high risk of mortality.

Serotonin Selective Re-uptake Inhibitors (SSRIs) are as effective as TCA in most patients, but with fewer side effects. They are also much safer in overdose. There has been little evidence to suggest routine TDM is helpful. There are other newer antidepressants contributing to the now minimal use of TCA.

This section will be illustrated with a typical TCA – amitriptyline, an SSRI – fluoxetine and lithium.

Amitriptyline

Clinical Use

IMPORTANT FACTS

- Tricyclic antidepressant
- One of the earliest successful drugs for treating depression
- Blocks serotonin and noradrenaline reuptake in the brain
- Active metabolite, nortriptyline, more selective for inhibition of noradrenaline uptake

Pharmacokinetics

IMPORTANT FACTS

- Metabolised to an equipotent desmethyl metabolite, nortriptyline
- Extensively metabolised
- Large volume of distribution
- Pharmacogenetic influences on metabolic clearance

Amitriptyline is extensively metabolised to desmethyl and hydroxyl metabolites.

The mono-desmethyl metabolite nortriptyline is pharmacologically active, the 10-hydroxy metabolite is not, nor are the di-desmethyl or other metabolites that are subsequently glucuronidated. Metabolism is influenced by CYP2D6 genotype (see Chapter 5) as well as self-induction of metabolism or induction by other drugs. The structure of amitriptyline is not dissimilar to chlorpromazine and it has similar pharmacokinetic properties.

SUMMARY OF AMITRIPTYLINE PHARMACOKINETICS

Parameter	Amitriptyline
Oral bioavailability (F)	~ 0.4
Fraction excreted renally	< 0.01
Fraction bound to plasma proteins	~ 0.95
Clearance (corrected for bioavailability) (mL/min/kg)	~ 11.5
Volume of distribution V_d (L/kg)	~ 15
Elimination half-life (h)	~ 20
Time to maximum concentration (h)	2 - 4

Toxicity
Anticholinergic side effects: dry mouth, urine retention, hypotension. The metabolites tend to accumulate in cardiac tissue and presumably contribute to the cardiotoxicity of this and other TCAs. As with phenothiazines, idiosyncratic toxic reactions occur rarely.

Monitoring therapy
Infrequently practiced in the UK, the target range is considered to be 50 - 150 µg/L. The nortriptyline metabolite should also be measured and the summed target range of 80 - 250 µg/L used.

Fluoxetine

Clinical use

IMPORTANT FACTS

- Used to treat depression and obsessive-compulsive disorder

- Can be used in children
- Also used to treat bulimia and premenstrual dysphoric disorder

Pharmacokinetics

IMPORTANT FACTS

- Prescribed as a racemate
- Desmethyl metabolite, norfluoxetine, pharmacologically active
- Long half-life; norfluoxetine up to 4 times longer
- Multiple CYP isoenzyme elimination
- Fluoxetine inhibits CYP2C9, the nor-metabolite also inhibits CYP3A4

Fluoxetine is well, if slowly, absorbed with a long elimination half-life, however the desmethyl metabolite as well as being pharmacologically active has a significantly longer half-life; the consequence is that steady state can take over a month to achieve. The long half-lives can enable the use of once weekly dosing. The inhibition of CYP2C9 results in increased phenytoin concentrations, the norfluoxetine inhibition of CYP3A4 may result in increased carbamazepine concentrations. The nor-metabolite is equipotent with the parent drug.

SUMMARY OF FLUOXETINE PHARMACOKINETICS

Parameter	Fluoxetine
Oral bioavailability (F)	~ 0.7
Fraction excreted renally	< 0.05
Fraction bound to plasma proteins	~ 0.95
Clearance (corrected for bioavailability) (mL/min/kg)	~ 10
Volume of distribution V_d (L/kg)	12 - 40
Elimination half-life (h) – fluoxetine	24 - 96
norfluoxetine	170 - 360
Time to maximum concentration (h)	6 - 8

Toxicity

As an SSRI fluoxetine is much less dangerous in overdose compared to a TCA. The inhibitory effects on CYP isoenzymes are noted above.

Monitoring therapy

- There is no evidence monitoring is useful

Although there appears to be a curvilinear relationship between plasma concentration and effect the need for therapeutic monitoring is not yet established.

Lithium

Clinical Use

IMPORTANT FACTS

- Identified serendipitously in the 1950s as an effective agent for bipolar disorder
- The exact mechanism of the mode of action of lithium has still not been conclusively elucidated.
- Modulates neurotransmission

Lithium carbonate is the usual form for oral administration – although other lithium salts can be used the carbonate is more stable. There is significant inter-individual variation in achieved serum concentrations on the same dose, this necessitates dose individualisation guided by repetitive monitoring.

Pharmacokinetics

IMPORTANT FACTS

- Administered orally
- A standardised sampling time of 12 hours post-dose is used
- Lithium does not bind to plasma proteins
- Distribution is even throughout body water
- Elderly have a 25% lower volume of distribution
- Lithium is renally excreted; reabsorption (cf. sodium) delays elimination
- Renal impairment can thus result in toxicity

Lithium absorption is dependent on the rate of dissolution and bioavailability, these factors can vary significantly between individuals. Distribution is throughout the body water, but with greater accumulation in brain, kidney, thyroid; pharmacokinetically lithium exhibits a two compartment open model.

In addition to the decreased clearance in the elderly there is also increased sensitivity. Lithium competes with sodium in the renal tubules for reabsorption, consequently factors affecting renal blood flow e.g. dehydration can cause detrimental accumulation. As with GFR there is a diurnal variation in lithium clearance, reflected in part by changes in posture.

SUMMARY OF LITHIUM PHARMACOKINETICS

Parameter	Lithium
Oral bioavailability (F)	1.0
Fraction excreted renally	1.0
Fraction bound to plasma proteins	0
Clearance (corrected for bioavailability) (mL/min/kg)	0.25 - 0.45
Volume of distribution V_d (L/kg)	0.5 - 0.8
Elimination half-life (h)	10 - 35
Time to maximum concentration (h)	2 - 4

Toxicity
The biggest single risk of toxicity is declining renal function. Nephrogenic diabetes insipidus is a recognised consequence of chronic lithium therapy, this is apparently due to lithium accumulation in the renal tubules; this effect is independent of the serum level and may occur even if the serum concentrations are maintained in the target range. Drug interactions with diuretics and other drugs all have their root cause in the impact of the drugs on renal sodium handling and consequently on lithium. Long-term lithium therapy is associated with hypothyroidism and may rarely be associated with hyperparathyroidism.

Monitoring therapy
Acute therapy for bipolar disorder may require plasma concentrations up to 1.2 mmol/L, though maintenance therapy would call for a maximum of 0.8 mmol/L. Relapses are more likely below 0.5 mmol/L. The higher the concentration the greater the side effects. As noted above a standardised sampling time of 12 hours post-dose in steady state is utilised. There have been attempts to relate efficacy to erythrocyte lithium concentrations, but this remains a research tool. Predictive tables using loading dose have been used to rapidly achieve a desired steady state concentration.

Structures of some antidepressants

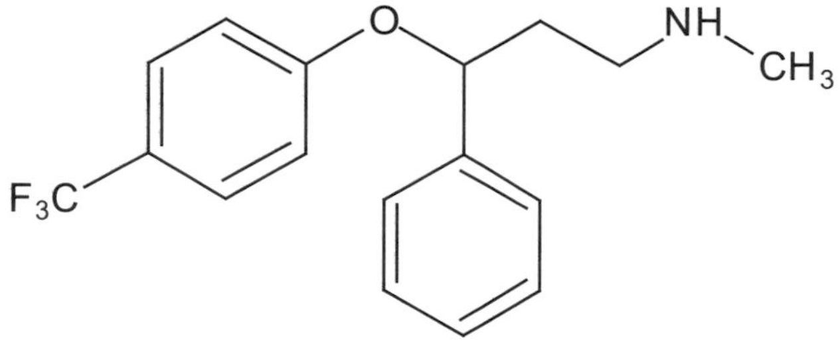

Fluoxetine

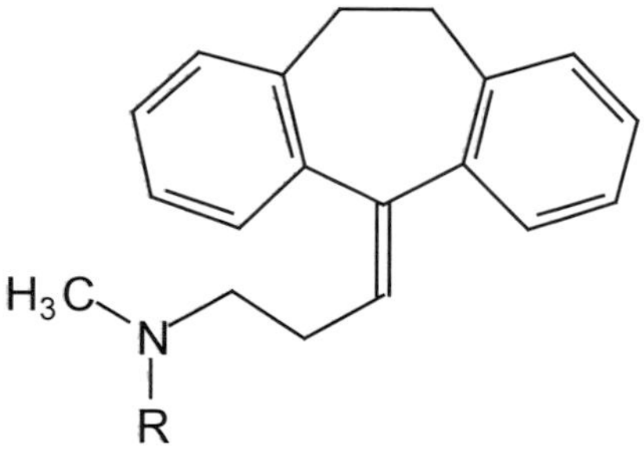

	R
Amitriptyline	CH$_3$
Nortriptyline	H

ANTIPSYCHOTICS

Chlorpromazine

Clinical Use

IMPORTANT FACTS

- First effective drug therapy used for schizophrenia

- 'Typical' antipsychotic
- Decreases agitation
- Is a member of the phenothiazine family of drugs

Chlorpromazine (CPZ) modifies the delusional, hallucinatory, hyperexcitable symptoms of schizophrenia. Although an old drug, introduced in the 1950s and with unpleasant side effects it is still in use today. Many other phenothiazines have been synthesised since. TDM is infrequently performed.

Pharmacokinetics

IMPORTANT FACTS

- Extensively metabolised
- Pharmacologically active metabolites
- Large volume of distribution

CPZ is readily absorbed after an oral dose. It is extensively metabolised with mono- and di-demethylation, N- and S-oxidation and 7-hydroxylation; there are also combinations of these e.g. 7-hydroxy di-*N*-desmethyl chlorpromazine; some of these metabolites have pharmacological activity and there is subsequent glucuronidation. The principal cytochrome P450 isoenzymes involved in metabolism are CYP1A2, 2D6 and 3A4. The large V_d means there is a very lengthy terminal elimination phase principally of low levels of metabolites; these may be detected many months after cessation of therapy.

SUMMARY OF CHLORPROMAZINE PHARMACOKINETICS

Parameter	Chlorpromazine
Oral bioavailability (F)	~ 0.3
Fraction excreted renally	< 0.01
Fraction bound to plasma proteins	~ 0.97
Clearance (corrected for bioavailability) (mL/min/kg)	~ 8.5
Volume of distribution V_d (L/kg)	~ 20
Elimination half-life (h)	~ 25
Time to maximum concentration (h)	2 - 4

Toxicity

Autonomic side effects: dry mouth, blurred vision, impotence. Orthostatic hypotension, idiosyncratic reactions occur rarely. Neurotoxicity is said to be associated with concentrations above 750 µg/L (2400 nmol/L). Deaths from overdose of chlorpromazine are rare and are associated with massive overdoses.

Monitoring therapy

Not routinely performed, target range is between 30 - 500 µg/L (94-1600 nmol/L).

Haloperidol

Clinical Use

IMPORTANT FACTS

- Effective in schizophrenia
- Serious side effects
- 'Typical' antipsychotic

The low doses used make investigation of its concentration-effect profile difficult.

Pharmacokinetics

IMPORTANT FACTS

- Readily absorbed orally
- Cleared by hepatic metabolism
- The reduced metabolite is also pharmacologically active

Haloperidol is well absorbed and metabolised by reduction of the ketone group to a secondary alcohol and to an N-dealkylated product. The cytochrome P450 isoenzymes involved are the same as for chlorpromazine; the reduced metabolite is the product of a ketone reductase whilst CYP2D6 back-converts it. The reduced metabolite has around 20% of the activity of the parent compound, but a longer half-life ~ 70h; this extended half-life reflects on-going conversion from haloperidol. Due to the cyclical nature of the metabolism of the reduced metabolite, CYP2D6 phenotype is important as poor metabolisers can have up to four times the concentration of the reduced metabolite when compared with extensive metabolisers.

Summary of haloperidol pharmacokinetics

Parameter	Haloperidol
Oral bioavailability (F)	0.4 - 0.8
Fraction excreted renally	< 0.01
Fraction bound to plasma proteins	~ 0.9
Clearance (corrected for bioavailability) (mL/min/kg)	12
Volume of distribution V_d (L/kg)	18
Elimination half-life (h)	~ 20
Time to maximum concentration (h)	1.7

Toxicity

Important Facts

- Extra-pyramidal side effects
- Tardive dyskinesia, may be irreversible after the drug is stopped

Symptoms typically take up to two years to develop and can persist indefinitely. Also see general comments on toxicity of antipsychotic drugs below.

Monitoring therapy

The target range for haloperidol is 1.5 - 5 µg/L (4 - 13 nmol/L), the relationship with the reduced metabolite is less clear, but confirmation that it is not accumulating excessively is appropriate if the dose is incremented.

Clozapine

Clinical use

Important Facts

- 'Atypical' antipsychotic
- Used in patients unresponsive to 'Typical' antipsychotics
- Risk of agranulocytosis
- Dose increased gradually

• Therapeutic effect may take weeks or months to occur

Clozapine is used in patients in whom other antipsychotics have failed. In this group around 40% will respond, hence its continued use despite the potentially life-threatening risk of neutropenia/agranulocytosis in ~ 3% of patients. Treatment initiation requires commencing with a low dose of 25 mg/day or less, and increasing this gradually to a maintenance dose of ten or twenty times this, meanwhile monitoring white cell counts. Use of an approved monitoring service is mandatory in the UK.

Pharmacokinetics

IMPORTANT FACTS

• Cleared by metabolism
• Wide (50-fold) variation in population metabolic clearance
• Pharmacologically active metabolites

Clozapine is metabolised through N-demethylation, N-oxidation and hydroxylation; these can occur in combination. Norclozapine (N-demethyl-clozapine) may be pharmacologically active and has a slightly longer half-life than clozapine, 20 hours versus 15 hours. Some of the N-oxide metabolite is recycled by reduction to clozapine. There is a dose/concentration relationship to both therapeutic effect and some side effects such as seizures and sedation. The main cytochrome P450 isoenzymes involved in metabolism are CYP1A2 and CYP3A4. In steady state the typical ratio of clozapine to norclozapine is ~ 1.32.

SUMMARY OF CLOZAPINE PHARMACOKINETICS

Parameter	Clozapine
Oral bioavailability (F)	~ 0.3
Fraction excreted renally	< 0.01
Fraction bound to plasma proteins	~ 0.96
Clearance (corrected for bioavailability) (mL/min/kg)	~ 6
Volume of distribution V_d (L/kg)	2.5 - 10
Elimination half-life (h)	8 - 16
Time to maximum concentration (h)	~ 2

Toxicity

IMPORTANT FACTS

- Neutropenia/agranulocytosis in ~ 3% of patients
- Variety of side effects
- Administration of a standard maintenance dose to a naïve individual is potentially fatal.

Neutropenia which may progress to agranulocytosis occurs unpredictably in 2-3% of patients. Doses must be escalated slowly on initiation of therapy as a standard maintenance dose is potentially fatal in a naïve subject causing hypotension, renal failure, seizures, tachycardia and coma. Side effects encountered in therapy include: headache, drowsiness, dizziness, sedation, tremor, weight gain, hypersalivation, seizures, tachycardia, hypotension; some of these are dose related.

Monitoring therapy

IMPORTANT FACTS

- Monitor both clozapine and its nor-metabolite
- Target concentration for clozapine is ~ 350 µg/L (~1100 nmol/L)
- Clozapine/norclozapine ratio in steady state is ~1.32

Extensive studies at the Medical Toxicology Unit in London have shown that a target clozapine concentration of ~ 350 µg/L (~1100 nmol/L) is consistent with optimal therapeutic effect. With a clozapine:norclozapine ratio of 1.32 the concomitant norclozapine concentration should be ~ 270 µg/L (~800 nmol/L). These are trough concentrations. The 'smoothing' effect of metabolism means there is less variation in the nor-concentration at other times post-dose and monitoring of the norclozapine concentration alone has been suggested, but not validated.

Adherence (compliance) with medication is a particularly important issue in this patient group; failure to medicate can have catastrophic consequences and has resulted in murder committed by the patient. Use of clozapine/norclozapine ratios can be used as an indication of adherence. In the London Unit's experience 2% samples sent for analysis have no detectable drug in them. Smoking enhances clearance and the SSRI fluvoxamine can inhibit clozapine metabolism. Younger patients also metabolise the drug faster and weight also needs to be considered. Women achieve plasma concentrations roughly 25% higher than men on the same dose; for these reasons a dosing nomogram is used.

General issues in TDM of anti-psychotic drugs

Mode of Action

Anti-psychotic drugs share properties and act through binding with dopamine and other receptors. There is insufficient space to discuss the neuroleptic, motor and extrapyramidal effects of the typical versus atypical agents. Drugs falling under the category of anti-psychotics include:

Phenothiazines
Chlorpromazine
Mesoridazine
Fluphenazine
Thioridazine
Trifluoperazine
Perphenazine

Thioxanthenes
Chlorprothixene
Thiothixene

Others
Haloperidol
Clozapine
Olanzapine
Quetiapine
Risperidone
Aripiprazole

Toxicity
In addition to the compound-specific effects noted in toxicity above, there are five recognised types of common neurological side effects.

ACUTE DYSTONIA
Occurs just after introduction of the drug, with spasms of the tongue, face, back, oculogyric crises; differentiation from hysteria is demonstrated if there is response to anti-parkinsonian agents.

AKATHISIA
Strong feelings of distress or discomfort, often with a need to keep walking around. Responds to dose reduction, but may be confused with agitation prompting an increase in dose!

PARKINSONISM

There is slowing of movements leading to rigidity, flat facies. Anti-parkinsonian agents are effective.

NEUROLEPTIC MALIGNANT SYNDROME

Is a rare presentation with severe Parkinsonian symptoms with stupor, fever, hyperthermia, unstable haemodynamics and rhabdomyolysis and consequent renal failure. This is a medical emergency; mortality may be as high as 10%.

TARDIVE DYSKINESIA

Occurs late in treatment in older patients. A stereotyped repetitive tic-like movement which may be associated with athetosis and potentially disabling dystonia. Clozapine is least likely to cause tardive dyskinesia and switching to this agent may bring relief.

Structures of some antipsychotic drugs

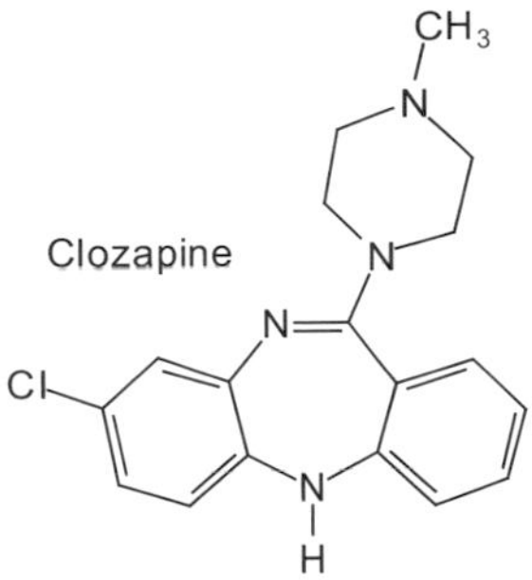

Clozapine

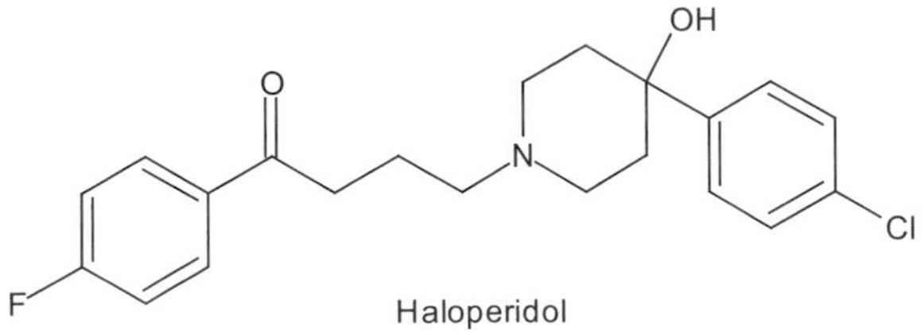

Haloperidol

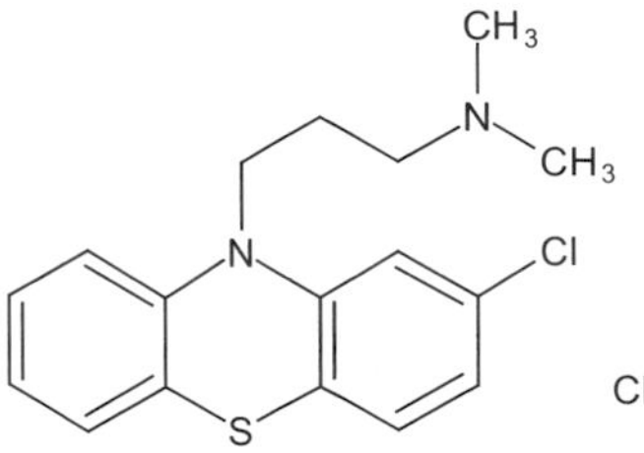

Chlorpromazine

BRONCHODILATOR DRUGS

Theophylline and caffeine

Clinical use

Theophylline and the related methylxanthines, caffeine and theobromine, share several pharmacological actions with potential therapeutic applications. They relax smooth muscle, and can thus relieve or prevent bronchoconstriction. They also stimulate the central nervous system, stimulate cardiac muscle and act on the kidney to produce a diuresis.

Theophylline is used for asthma and stable chronic obstructive pulmonary disease. The advent of more effective and less toxic adrenoceptor agonists and anticholinergic bronchodilators has meant that theophylline is no longer a first- or second-line drug in chronic asthma, but it is still useful in small children and elderly patients who have difficulty with inhalers, and in patients with predominantly nocturnal symptoms.

Caffeine is used in neonates to treat apnoea of prematurity, having taken over from theophylline in this setting, as dose regimes are simpler and the effects are more predictable.

Pharmacokinetics

Theophylline is completely and rapidly absorbed from liquids and uncoated tablets, with peak concentrations occurring within 1 - 2 hours of a single oral dose on an empty stomach. Peak concentrations are delayed up to 6 - 8 hours post-dose after food or if sustained release preparations are used. Intravenous preparations of theophylline generally contain aminophylline, which is the ethylene diamine salt and is more soluble. Aminophylline preparations are approximately 80% theophylline by weight, and this must be taken into account in pharmacokinetic calculations and estimation of equivalent doses.

IMPORTANT FACTS

- Methylxanthines are metabolised in the liver
- Theophylline is metabolised by hydroxylation to 1,3 dimethyluric acid, then demethylation to 1-methyluric acid
- Other methylated xanthines are also formed
- Rate of metabolism is affected by a large number of factors – hepatic disease, other drugs, dietary factors, smoking etc.
- Plasma theophylline concentrations are increased in heart failure, cirrhosis and viral infections, and decreased in smokers, chronic alcoholics and by

drugs that induce hepatic metabolism
- Caffeine is metabolised in adults by oxidation and demethylation to 1-methylxanthine and 1-methyluric acid
- Caffeine elimination is prolonged in neonates due to immaturity of cytochrome P450 1A2. Parent drug is predominantly excreted renally in the first three months of life

SUMMARY OF THEOPHYLLINE PHARMACOKINETICS

Parameter	Theophylline	Caffeine
Oral bioavailability (F)	> 0.95	> 0.95
Fraction excreted renally	0.1	0.85
Fraction bound to plasma proteins	0.5 - 0.65	0.3 - 0.4
Clearance (corrected for bioavailability) (mL/min/kg)	0.5	0.1 - 0.17
Volume of distribution V_d (L/kg)	0.4 - 0.6	0.9
Elimination half-life (h)	3 - 9	40 - 230
Time to maximum concentration (h) (im/iv)	2.0	

Toxicity
Side effects are relatively frequent with theophylline – mild or moderate effects such as nausea, headache and jitteriness are common within the 'target range' (see below) and more serious effects (tremor, agitation, insomnia, diarrhoea, palpitations, cardiac arrhythmias and seizures) occur with increasing frequency at plasma concentrations above 20 mg/L (110 μmol/L).

Caffeine produces much less tachycardia and fewer fits than theophylline, and toxicity is less of a problem overall.

Monitoring therapy
The variation in the rate of metabolism of methylxanthines accounts for the poor correlation between dose and plasma concentration, justifying the role of therapeutic drug monitoring. The relationship between plasma theophylline concentration and effect (forced expiratory volume in the first second, FEV1) is linear over the range 3 - 20 mg/L (17 - 110 μmol/L). However, improvements in FEV1 at concentrations below 10 mg/L (55 μmol/L) are often small, and the lower limit of the therapeutic range is often set around this figure. Some patients undoubtedly show a useful response at lower plasma concentrations. Other factors such

as mucosal thickening and plugging of the airways are not responsive to theophylline, and may obscure the relationship between concentration and effect. The therapeutic range for theophylline is normally taken as 10 - 20 mg/L (55 - 110 µmol/L).

Concentration monitoring for theophylline is useful in initial dosage optimisation, particularly as the wide pharmacokinetic variation means that published dosage recommendations tend to be conservative. A steady state trough concentration is usually the best and most reproducible parameter for monitoring. Concentration measurements are also of undoubted value in confirming theophylline toxicity and monitoring the overdosed patient, and if aminophylline is to be given to patients who have been taking oral theophylline preparations. Non-adherence with therapy is common, but the variable pharmacokinetics mean that it is not always easy to assess with concentration measurements.

In neonates with apnoea, caffeine concentrations in the range 5 - 20 mg/L (25 - 100 µmol/L) are generally associated with improved respiration. The lower toxicity and more predictable pharmacokinetics combine to reduce the need for therapeutic monitoring, and a cost-effective rationale has not yet been established.

Structures of theophylline and caffeine

Theophylline   Caffeine

CARDIOACTIVE DRUGS

Amiodarone

Clinical use

IMPORTANT FACTS

- Treatment should be initiated and normally monitored only under hospital or specialist supervision
- Indicated only for the treatment of severe rhythm disorders not responding to other therapies or when other treatments cannot be used, specifically:
  - tachyarrhythmias associated with Wolff-Parkinson-White Syndrome
  - atrial flutter and fibrillation when other drugs cannot be used
  - all types of tachyarrhythmias of paroxysmal nature including: supra-ventricular, nodal and ventricular tachycardias, ventricular fibrillation: when other drugs cannot be used

Amiodarone is a structural analogue of thyroxine and some of its anti-arrhythmic properties and toxicity may be due to interactions with thyroid hormone receptors. It was originally developed for the treatment of angina but since the mid 1970s the drug has been used in the treatment of ventricular tachyarrhythmias. Although considered to be a class III anti-arrhythmic, amiodarone also has class I, II and IV actions, which gives it a unique pharmacological profile.

Amiodarone has a very large volume of distribution and when given orally takes days to suppress ventricular tachyarrhythmias. However, intravenous amiodarone has an immediate effect and can be used in life-threatening ventricular arrhythmias. Often survivors of myocardial infarction (MI) die during the subsequent year; this is thought to be due to ventricular arrhythmia. In patients with preserved cardiac function amiodarone reduces sudden death after MI. The drug can also prevent the sudden cardiac death, predominantly due to ventricular arrhythmias, which often occur in patients with heart failure.

When given orally, amiodarone's large volume of distribution requires the use of a loading dose in order that therapeutically effective plasma concentrations are reached relatively quickly. The oral loading dose is 200 mg given three times a day for a week, followed by 200 mg twice a day for a further week. The maintenance dose is 200 mg once a day or the minimum dose that controls the arrhythmia.

Used intravenously for the suppression of arrhythmias, the drug is administered via the caval vein as a 5 mg/kg infusion over 20 minutes to 2 hours with ECG monitoring of efficacy. Further infusions can be given if necessary up to a maximum dose of 1200 mg. Intravenous use of the drug can also be called for during cardiopulmonary resuscitation; in this indication 300 mg is given as a short, < 3 minute, infusion after the administration of adrenaline to treat ventricular fibrillation or pulseless tachycardia that is refractory to defibrillation.

Amiodarone has proved effective in reducing sudden cardiac death in patients with Chagas' disease. This disease is caused by a protozoan parasite, *Trypanosoma cruzi*, which is transmitted to humans through the faeces of infected bloodsucking insects that are endemic in certain areas of Latin America. The parasite causes a cardiac myopathy which may only appear decades after the initial infection and causes life threatening cardiac arrhythmias. In addition to its therapeutic action in preventing cardiac arrhythmias, amiodarone has been shown to have direct activity against *Trypanosoma cruzi*, both *in vitro* and *in vivo*.

Pharmacokinetics

IMPORTANT FACTS

- Very lipid soluble, log octanol/water partition coefficient ~ 6.7
- Volume of distribution ~ 5000 L
- Elimination half-life ~ 50 days
- Active metabolite, mono-N-desethylamiodarone
- There are several clinically significant pharmacokinetic drug interactions

Amiodarone has a very high octanol/water partition coefficient and consequently the drug is distributed extensively into tissues. This results in an apparent volume of distribution in excess of 5000 litres. When administered orally the drug has an oral bioavailability of between 20 and 80%. The drug is extensively metabolised during its first pass through the liver where it is de-ethylated to the primary, active, metabolite mono-N-desethylamiodarone. This metabolite is even more lipid soluble than the parent compound. Peak blood concentrations are reached 3 to 7 hours after ingestion and the drug is highly protein bound to albumin and β-lipoprotein.

The extremely large volume of distribution and long plasma half-life of amiodarone make precise estimation of the pharmacokinetic parameters difficult. Early estimates of the drug's half-life were as low as 18 hours and resulted from low assay sensitivity and inadequately short sampling times. In addition, there are other unique aspects of the drug's disposition kinetics that result from its extremely high lipid solubility.

Amiodarone is a potent inhibitor of the metabolism of several drugs. The drug inhibits metabolism by several cytochrome P450 pathways, including CYP2C9 (metabolises warfarin), CYP2D6 (metabolises several beta-blockers, codeine and morphine), and CYP3A4 (which metabolises many drugs). Interactions with warfarin, digoxin and simvastatin are the most clinically important.

Amiodarone reduces warfarin clearance causing pronounced increases in the prothrombin time and International Normalised Ratio (INR). This interaction may take some time to reach maximum and requires frequent monitoring of the INR until stabilised.

Digoxin plasma concentrations predictably double after coadministration with amiodarone. The increase occurs because of the inhibition of digoxin secretion by the renal tubules and the inhibition of the P-glycoprotein membrane transporter system. Hence the dose of digoxin should be reduced by 50% when amiodarone is started, and plasma digoxin concentrations should be monitored closely.

There is an increased incidence of myopathy and/or rhabdomyolysis when simvastatin dosage is higher than 20 mg/day. Simvastatin is metabolised primarily by CYP3A4 and, since amiodarone is an inhibitor of this enzyme, the interaction is likely to be related to the increased simvastatin concentrations. It should be borne in mind that in the UK simvastatin is available without prescription over the counter (OTC) at pharmacies. Amiodarone metabolism and plasma concentrations may be affected by inhibitors of metabolism such as cimetidine and grapefruit juice.

SUMMARY OF AMIODARONE PHARMACOKINETICS

Parameter	Amiodarone
Oral bioavailability (F)	0.65
Fraction excreted renally	0
Fraction bound to plasma proteins	> 0.98
Clearance (corrected for bioavailability) (mL/min/kg)	1.9
Volume of distribution V_d (L/kg)	70
Elimination half-life (d)	50
Time to maximum concentration (h)	4.5

Toxicity

IMPORTANT FACTS

- Toxicity is related to dosage and duration of treatment
- Most serious adverse effect is pulmonary toxicity
- Thyroid toxicity is the most common complication
- Can cause the visible extremities of patients to turn blue

The most serious adverse effect of amiodarone therapy is pulmonary toxicity, which can result from amiodarone-induced phospholipidosis or immune-mediated hypersensitivity. The usual clinical manifestation is cough and progressive difficulty in breathing (dyspnoea), with associated patchy interstitial infiltrates on chest radiographs and reduced diffusing capacity on lung function tests. In extreme cases patients may present with adult respiratory distress syndrome (ARDS). In most instances, the toxicity is reversible with the primary treatment being withdrawal of amiodarone, supportive care and, if required, corticosteroids. Thyroid abnormalities/toxicity may occur in around 10 percent of patients receiving long-term amiodarone therapy. Hyperthyroidism may result from an excess of iodine or acute thyroiditis, but hypothyroidism is two to four times more common than hyperthyroidism. If appropriate, both can be reversed by amiodarone withdrawal. However, if the drug cannot be withdrawn safely then appropriate therapy can be used to reverse the hyper- or hypothyroid state.

Cardiac toxicity, bradycardia and heart block, occur in a small proportion of patients (< 3%), as does liver toxicity (< 1%) and neurotoxicity (< 0.5%). Photosensitivity is common in patients receiving amiodarone therapy and all patients should be cautioned to use sun block to cover exposed skin when they are outdoors. Failure to do so causes bluish skin discolouration, thought to be due to the iodine in amiodarone, to develop on exposed areas. Microdeposits are visible on slit-lamp examination of the cornea in nearly all patients treated with the drug. However, they rarely affect vision. Discontinuation of the drug resolves both the skin discoloration and the corneal deposits after several months.

Monitoring therapy

IMPORTANT FACTS

- Complicated by the drug's extreme pharmacokinetics
- Both the parent drug and its metabolite, mono-N-desethylamiodarone, should be measured
- The recommended sampling time is pre-dose

Although many of the drug's adverse effects are dose/concentration-related there is not a need for therapeutic drug monitoring in the majority of patients. Below amiodarone concentrations of 0.5 mg/L (0.8 µmol/L) in plasma the drug shows little anti-arrhythmic action and adverse reactions are commonly seen in patients with plasma concentrations > 2.5 mg/L (3.8 µmol/L). So, in some patients, monitoring plasma amiodarone concentrations may differentiate failure of drug therapy from suboptimal dosing or poor adherence, while in others it may reduce the incidence of concentration-related side effects. However, it should be noted that the pulmonary side effects of the drug may occur at plasma amiodarone concentrations < 2.5 mg/L (3.8 µmol/L).

Amiodarone concentrations are relatively easy to measure by high performance liquid chromatography (HPLC). However, any analytical method used to measure amiodarone should be able to measure not only the parent drug, but also the primary metabolite mono-N-desethylamiodarone. In most patients at steady state these two compounds will be found at very similar concentrations. During long term therapy if samples are assayed in which the concentration of the parent drug greatly exceeds that of the metabolite then the possibility of poor adherence should be considered.

Digoxin

Clinical use

IMPORTANT FACTS

- Used in the management of chronic cardiac failure where the dominant problem is systolic dysfunction.
- Its therapeutic benefit is greatest in those patients with ventricular dilatation.
- Specifically indicated where cardiac failure is accompanied by atrial fibrillation
- Used in the management of certain supraventricular arrhythmias, particularly chronic atrial flutter and fibrillation

In 1785 William Withering published *'An account of the foxglove and some of its medical uses'* in which he described his ten years of experience in the use of foxglove for the treatment of patients with dropsy. Although we no longer use the crude extract of foxglove in medicine, digoxin, the purified cardiac glycoside extracted from *digitalis larnata* (the yellow foxglove plant) is in widespread use over 220 years after Withering published his observations.

Digoxin's primary mechanism of action comes from its ability to bind to a site on the extracellular aspect of the α-subunit of the sodium-potassium ATPase pump in the membranes of cardiac myocytes. This inhibits the pump and causes an increase in the intracellular concentration of sodium ions, which then leads to a rise in the concentration of calcium ions. The increased amounts of calcium are then available to the contractile proteins and this increases the force of myocardial contraction. The inhibition of the sodium-potassium pump is also thought to improve the sensitivity of the baroreceptors. The drug also increases vagal activity via its central action on the central nervous system; this slows the conduction of electrical impulses through the atrioventricular (AV) node. This increases the refractory period of the AV node and is important for digoxin's clinical use in the management of certain supraventricular arrhythmias.

For the treatment of heart failure, the evidence base from clinical trial data shows that digoxin therapy is most beneficial in patients with enlarged hearts, poor pump function, and low ejection fractions. Digoxin is unlikely to benefit patients with a high risk of cardiac failure due to comorbidities such as hypertension, diabetes or hyperlipidemia; or those patients with asymptomatic structural heart disease. In these patients, it is important to first reduce the risk factors and then initiate therapy with ACE inhibitors and β-blockers, if indicated. In such patients, digoxin should be reserved for symptomatic patients treated with diuretics and ACE inhibitors with or without β-blockers.

Digoxin is usually given orally, but can also be given by intravenous infusion if the clinical situation warrants it. For rapid digitalisation 1 to 1.5 mg is given orally in divided doses for the first 24 hours. If the need is less urgent then the initial dose is 250 to 500 µg orally. For emergency treatment the drug can be given as an intravenous infusion of 0.75 to 1 mg over at least two hours. The maintenance dose is 62.5 to 500 µg/day orally and depends on heart rate response when given for atrial fibrillation.

Digoxin is eliminated renally, so extra care should be taken in patients with impaired renal function and in the elderly.

Digoxin is a critical dose drug; so small changes in dose can result in either loss of efficacy or serious adverse effects. There are several examples in the literature of bioequivalence differing between healthy volunteers and patients. For this reason it may be important that patients are maintained on the same formulation, so digoxin should be prescribed by the proprietary brand name and not generically.

Pharmacokinetics

IMPORTANT FACTS

- Mainly eliminated via the kidneys
- Nearly all plasma concentration measurements have been made by immunoassay
- Digoxin is a substrate for P-glycoprotein
- There are clinically significant pharmacokinetic drug interactions

Since the volume of distribution of digoxin is relatively high, around 7 L/kg, and the dose of the drug is low, typically 125 µg/day, the peak plasma concentrations of digoxin are low, < 5 µg/L (< 6.4 nmol/L). In addition the molecular weight of digoxin is 781 daltons and the melting point is 249°C. These factors make the drug difficult to analyse at the concentrations that occur in plasma by most techniques, except accelerator mass spectrometer (AMS), very sensitive high performance liquid chromatography – tandem mass spectrometry (HPLC-MS/MS) or immunoassay. Since digoxin is an old drug and HPLC-MS/MS and AMS have only recently become available, all the pharmacokinetic data have been derived using data derived from immunoassays or radioisotope studies, and may have, at least in part, been contaminated by cross reactions with metabolites and digoxin-like immunoreactive substances (DLIS).

Many drugs produce clinically significant pharmacokinetic interactions with digoxin and digoxin interaction studies are often part of new drug development. Drugs that decrease the plasma digoxin concentration by decreasing absorption include antacids, cholestyramine, and dietary fibre. Drugs that decrease the plasma digoxin concentration by increasing non-renal clearance include enzyme inducers such as rifampicin and phenytoin. St John's wort also reduces plasma digoxin concentrations, by about 25%, and this may be due to a combined action of reducing absorption by induction of CYP3A4 and/or P-glycoprotein in the gut and increased metabolism in the liver by CYP3A4.

Certain antibiotics, including neomycin and aminosalicylic acid, reduce digoxin absorption while others, including erythromycin, clarithromycin and tetracycline, increase the bioavailability of digoxin in some patients. The increase in digoxin concentrations is thought to be due to inactivation of bacterial metabolism in the intestines. Changing intestinal motility also affects digoxin absorption; reducing motility by coadministration of diphenoxylate (Lomotil) or propantheline increases absorption whereas metoclopramide, which increases motility, reduces digoxin absorption. Capsule preparations of digoxin in solution are less subject to several of these interactions which more frequently affect the bioavailability of digoxin from tablets.

Various drugs induce alterations in the volume of distribution and clearance of digoxin. Cardiac patients receiving digoxin therapy are particularly prone to interactions with commonly co-administered medications such as the antiar-rhythmics quinidine and amiodarone, the calcium channel blockers verapamil and nifedipine, and possibly some vasodilating agents.

SUMMARY OF DIGOXIN PHARMACOKINETICS

Parameter	Digoxin
Oral bioavailability (F)	0.7
Fraction excreted renally	0.6
Fraction bound to plasma proteins	0.25
Clearance (corrected for bioavailability) (mL/min/kg)	0.88 CrCl +0.33*
Volume of distribution V_d (L/kg)	7
Elimination half-life (h)	36
Time to maximum concentration (h)	1

*In patients with some degree of heart failure. CrCl = creatinine clearance in mL/min/kg.

Toxicity

IMPORTANT FACTS

- Toxicity is related to drug concentration, but is exacerbated by hypokalaemia
- Gastrointestinal adverse events include nausea, vomiting, diarrhoea or constipation and abdominal pain
- Neurotoxicity is manifest as headaches, fatigue, insomnia, confusion, or vertigo
- Visual disturbances are common with blurred vision, colour casts and coloured halos being classic signs of digoxin toxicity
- Cardiac toxicity is exhibited as bradycardia, atrioventricular block, ventricular tachycardias and other arrhythmias
- Serious intoxications can be treated with anti-digoxin antibody fragments (e.g. Digibind®)

The unwanted effects of digoxin are directly related to the concentration of the drug in plasma. However, measurement of digoxin concentrations alone is not sufficient as toxicity is increased if potassium concentrations are low. In addition, toxicity is related to the degree of heart disease present and the age of the patient. Advanced age is an independent risk factor in developing toxicity and toxicity is more likely to arise in those patients with serious heart disease. Toxicity can usually be reversed by withdrawing digoxin or reducing digoxin plasma concentrations and, when present, correcting the patient's hypokalaemia.

In the USA it has been estimated that around 0.4% of all hospital admissions are due to digoxin toxicity and that around 1% of outpatients on digoxin exhibit toxicity. In the elderly and infirm, such as nursing home patients, the incidence may be as high as 10 to 18%. However, the increased awareness of drug interactions and the decreased use of digoxin to treat heart failure and arrhythmias has reduced the incidence of digoxin toxicity.

The visual disturbances that arise from digoxin toxicity include the classic signs of yellow colour casts and halos being experienced by patients. This has led to the speculation that the painter Vincent van Gogh suffered from digitalis toxicity, possibly exacerbated by an interaction with the terpenes in absinthe. Some of van Gogh's most famous paintings are representative of the visual disturbances experienced by patients who have digoxin toxicity; for example several of his 'Sunflowers' pictures and the 'Chair' exhibit distinctly yellowish casts while 'The Starry Night' contains yellow halos around the stars.

Monitoring therapy

IMPORTANT FACTS

- Blood should be drawn pre-dose or at least 6 hours post-dose
- Both the plasma digoxin and potassium concentrations should be measured
- The occurrence of interference from DLIS should be borne in mind

Digoxin was one of the first drugs to be dosed according to plasma drug concentration and was a prototype for concentration guided dosing and the development of therapeutic drug monitoring. In the mid to late 1970s the traditional therapeutic range of 0.8 to 2.0 μg/L (1.0 - 2.6 nmol/L) was established; this was originally to minimise digoxin toxicity rather than to maximise efficacy. However, since then a number of outcome trials for the use of the drug have been carried out to determine the benefit of digoxin therapy in heart failure.

Retrospective subgroup analysis of the Digitalis Investigators Group trial (DIG) showed increased mortality in men at plasma digoxin concentrations > 1.0 µg/L (> 1.3 nmol/L) whereas there was decreased mortality at concentrations of 0.5 to 0.8 µg/L (0.6 - 1.0 nmol/L). Reanalysis of the PROVED (Prospective Randomized Study of Ventricular Failure and the Efficacy of Digoxin) and RADIANCE (Randomized Assessment of Digoxin on Inhibitors of the Angiotensin Converting Enzyme) trials indicated that the group of patients with plasma digoxin concentrations between 0.5 to 0.9 µg/L (0.6 - 1.2 nmol/L) experienced comparable benefits regarding symptoms of heart failure, improvement in LVEF, and increased treadmill time, compared with patient groups with plasma digoxin concentrations between 1.0 to 1.2 µg/L (1.3 - 1.5 nmol/L) or > 1.2 µg/L (> 1.5 nmol/L). The evidence suggest, therefore, that for the treatment of heart failure, the optimal plasma digoxin concentration target would be 0.7 µg/L (0.9 nmol/L) with the aim of keeping concentrations within the range 0.5 to 1.0 µg/L (0.6 - 1.3 nmol/L). This would minimise digoxin toxicity and maximise the drug's efficacy.

Endogenous substances that cross react with digoxin radioimmunoassays, digoxin-like immunoreactive substances (DLIS), occasionally yield spuriously high serum or plasma digoxin concentration measurements. DLIS is more prevalent in the blood of the very young, particularly neonates, and the elderly. Commercially available digoxin assays vary in their specificity to DLIS and their ability to distinguish DLIS from exogenous digoxin. The artificial elevation of a reported digoxin concentration can have very serious clinical consequences for patients and has resulted in erroneous malpractice accusations made against staff. The occurrence of DLIS should be considered if plasma digoxin concentrations are unexpectedly and inexplicably high.

Structures of amiodarone and digoxin

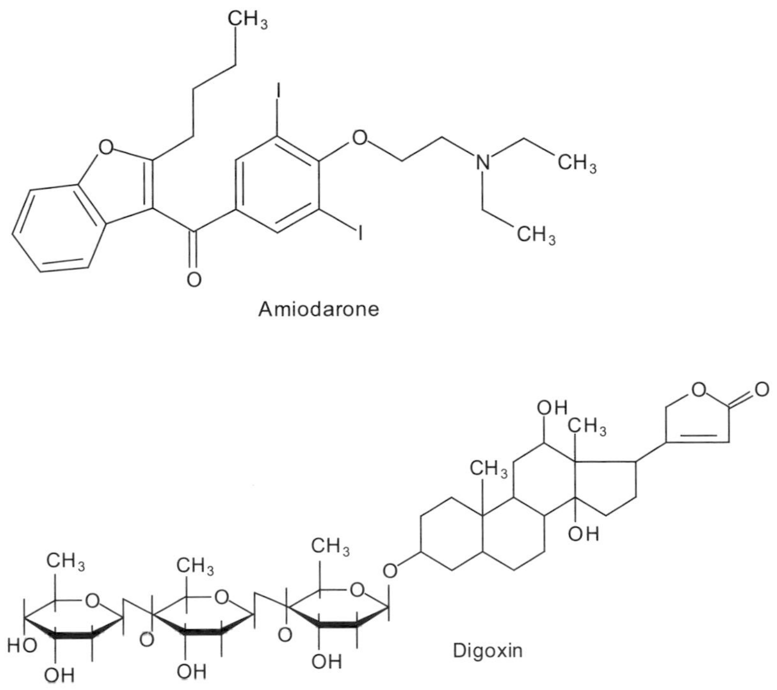

Amiodarone

Digoxin

DRUGS OF ABUSE

Drug abusers repetitively misuse and are addicted to this behaviour. While total abstinence is desirable, this is extremely difficult to achieve, particularly if the abuser is in a social context where the substance of choice is readily available. A chaotic lifestyle can develop as a characteristic of the irregular availability of supply and money to buy drugs. Harm reduction strategies require control of the chaos and substitute drugs are given to assuage the craving. Pharmacologically pure drugs are supplied to further reduce overdose and infection risks. While pure versions of the drug may be used this may have a non-ideal pharmacokinetic or effect profile. A substitute that blocks receptors, has a longer half-life and is less toxic is preferable. Substitutes may be subject to the variables of pharmacokinetics/dynamics as for any other drug and/or have a relatively low therapeutic index, with optimal concentrations for non-toxic effect i.e. therapeutic drug monitoring principles may be applicable.

A further issue is adherence, the question being are they taking the substitute? While detection in e.g. urine may provide confirmation, the more sophisticated question of what is the optimal dose in this individual requires quantitative measurement, typically in plasma. There has been much recent interest in dosage optimisation of substitutes, particularly those where the alleles of the metabolising enzyme could result in wide differences in concentration for the same dose. Monitoring allows rapid individualisation of substitute therapy and minimisation of untoward effects.

Methadone

Clinical use

IMPORTANT FACTS

- Is a long acting μ receptor agonist
- Administered as a racemate, the R-isomer has ~ 30 times more activity than the S-isomer as a μ receptor agonist
- Suppresses withdrawal symptoms in opioid addicted individuals
- Causes respiratory depression and sedation
- The R-isomer is an effective analgesic
- The S-isomer may have some immunosuppressive activity
- Can be lethal if too high a dose is given

Pharmacologically methadone has much in common with morphine. It binds to the μ receptor, hence its effectiveness as a morphine (main plasma metabolite of heroin) substitute. It can be given orally and is an effective analgesic and suppressant of opioid withdrawal symptoms. The analgesic effect is similar to morphine, but methadone has a longer half-life with the risk of accumulation if given repeatedly. Patients taking methadone develop tolerance to its effect necessitating the use of increasing doses. There is a risk that should they cease to take methadone for a period of time and then take their previous high dose they will have lost their tolerance and will suffer life-threatening toxicity. This is a not uncommon cause of death in this population.

Pharmacokinetics

IMPORTANT FACTS

- Rapidly absorbed after oral dosing
- Extensively metabolised
- Extensively distributed

• Phenytoin and rifampicin induce metabolism

About 90% of methadone is protein bound in plasma. It is rapidly absorbed after an oral dose and extensively metabolised; although the rate of excretion is affected by some other drugs e.g. phenytoin. It is more rapidly excreted in acid urine. The main metabolites are N-demethyl and, following ring cyclization, pyrrolidines and pyrroline. The principal metabolite of methadone is 2-ethylidene-1,5-dimethyl-3,3-diphenyl-pyrrolidine (EDDP).

There can be significant intra-individual variation in R-methadone concentrations. Methadone is metabolised stereoselectively, the R-isomer is preferentially metabolised by CYP2C19 and the S-isomer by CYP2B6. CYP3A4 has no role in methadone metabolism. The plasma half-lives of the R- and S-isomers are 37.5 h and 28.5 h and volumes of distribution are 500 L and 290 L in a 70 kg man respectively.

Drug interactions may be important, for example, the anti-retroviral drug nelfinavir reduces both R- and S-methadone concentrations.

SUMMARY OF METHADONE PHARMACOKINETICS

Parameter	Methadone
Oral bioavailability (F)	0.95
Fraction excreted renally	0.25
Fraction bound to plasma proteins	~ 0.9
Clearance (corrected for bioavailability) (mL/min/kg)	1.0 - 3.5
Volume of distribution V_d (L/kg)	~ 6.5
Elimination half-life (h)	15 - 40
Time to maximum concentration (h)	~ 4

Toxicity

IMPORTANT FACTS

• Respiratory depressant
• Vasodilatation causing hypotension

While there are many side effects from using opiates the most important toxic effect is respiratory depression. Overdose should be treated as for any opiate with opiate antagonists such as naloxone. The long half-life of methadone should be recognised and repeated doses of the antagonist may be required. Children are particularly susceptible to methadone poisoning.

Monitoring therapy

- Plasma methadone (total concentration) monitoring is adequate
- An acceptable range is 150 - 250 µg/L (430 - 720 nmol/L)
- Saliva/oral fluid monitoring requires further validation
- Presence of EDDP in urine is proof of ingestion and hence compliance

The use of therapeutic drug monitoring of total methadone indicates that there is a threshold concentration of 50 µg/L (140 nmol/L). Plasma concentrations need to be maintained above this threshold to avoid withdrawal symptoms, with an optimal concentration of around 150 - 250 µg/L (430 - 720 nmol/L). The relationship between effect and concentration is as good for total as for R-methadone, and hence the former is analysed as it is less analytically challenging. Attempts to monitor methadone concentrations using saliva have shown poor correlation with plasma values and salivary monitoring is not routinely recommended.

Routine practice in monitoring addicts on methadone therapy, is to confirm the presence of methadone and/or the metabolite EDDP in urine as proof of concordance. It is preferable to detect EDDP as this confirms metabolism. Addicts may 'spike' their urine with methadone to get a positive result, thereby 'confirming' adherance with therapy and thus ensuring a further prescription, which can be sold on to get cash to buy drugs of choice.

Buprenorphine

Clinical use

IMPORTANT FACTS

- Partial µ receptor agonist/antagonist
- Used in managing withdrawal from opiate dependency
- Analgesic

Buprenorphine has an effect profile similar to morphine, but is more potent by a factor of ~ 20. Analgesia is long lasting reflecting slow turnover at the µ receptor. Since the drug is a partial agonist, cessation of long-term therapy can result in moderate symptoms of withdrawal.

Comparisons with methadone of retention rate on therapy, rate of illicit opiate use and craving depend on the buprenorphine dose and regimen employed. Some studies claim 8 mg/day with high dose methadone (80 mg) to be more effective. Retention rates for the former may be influenced by slower induction of buprenorphine effect. Higher doses of buprenorphine are associated with decreasing *in vivo* μ receptor availability.

Pharmacokinetics

IMPORTANT FACTS

- Sublingual, intramuscular or intravenous administration
- Pharmacodynamics not correlated with plasma concentrations
- Norbuprenorphine is the main metabolite

Buprenorphine is satisfactorily absorbed by sub-lingual administration, though im or iv routes are also used. Buccal administration gives half the bioavailability of sub-lingual administration, which itself is about 50% bioavailable. The main phase one metabolite is norbuprenorphine through N-dealkylation by CYP3A4. This and other metabolites are conjugated. There is no significant renal excretion of the parent drug, but up to 30% of the dose is excreted renally as water soluble conjugates. The iv terminal half-life is shorter than following buccal or sub-lingual administration, probably reflecting an oral depot effect. The terminal half-life for buprenorphine is ~ 42 h while that of norbuprenorphine is ~ 57 h. Alternate day administration has been advocated to reflect the long terminal half-life.

Plasma concentrations of buprenorphine and its nor-metabolite show a dose dependency; concentrations above 0.7 μg/L (1.5 nmol/L) result in minimal withdrawal symptoms. Sub-lingual preparations are readily soluble and therefore easily abused by injection. To counter this naloxone has been added to some preparations; this does not affect buprenorphine kinetics. Concentrations up to 14 μg/L (30 nmol/L) have been recorded in breast milk; this would result in an insignificant dose to the baby.

Adherance testing using urine requires specific assays because 'opiate screen' immunoassays lack the ability to detect buprenorphine or its nor-metabolite. Since the metabolite is present at ~ 20-fold higher concentration than the parent drug it is the preferred target analyte.

Summary of buprenorphine pharmacokinetics

Parameter	Buprenorphine
Oral bioavailability (F)*	~ 0.5
Fraction excreted renally	< 0.01
Fraction bound to plasma proteins	0.96
Clearance (corrected for bioavailability) (mL/min/kg)	13
Volume of distribution V_d (L/kg)	1.5
Elimination half-life (h)	2.5 - 44
Time to maximum concentration (h)	0.5*
*sublingual	

Toxicity

Important Fact

- Buprenorphine in combination with benzodiazepines or other opiates may be fatal

Mortality studies in the UK and France indicate a low but definite level of deaths attributable to buprenorphine. Most deaths associated with buprenorphine had contributory factors, benzodiazepines or other drugs in particular.

Monitoring therapy

- Monitoring of plasma concentrations has not yet been validated
- Norbuprenorpine detectable in urine is proof of ingestion and hence compliance

Amfetamines

Clinical use

IMPORTANT FACTS

- Adrenergic agonists
- Amfetamines are racemic
- There are many analogues with different activity profiles

Amfetamines are powerful sympathomimetic CNS stimulants. They were used as appetite suppressants and still have a role in some disorders such as Attention Deficit Hyperactivity Disorder. Therapeutic treatment tends to administer pro-drugs such as selegiline. Adderall may also be used and is a 3:1 mixture of R/S salts.

Dexedrine (D-amfetamine) is used therapeutically in managing amfetamine users.

Therapeutic monitoring of amfetamines in serum is not established practice. Detection of L/D ratios has been used as a measure of adherance with D-amfetamine therapy and to differentiate legitimate D-amfetamine therapy from abuse of 'street' amfetamine, as the latter is usually a racemate.

Cocaine

Clinical Use

IMPORTANT FACTS

- Is used to create a blood-free operative field
- Local anaesthetic
- A stimulant typically snorted, smoked or injected

Detection of one of the cocaine metabolites benzoylecgonine or ecgonine methyl ester confirm use. Cocaine detection in saliva is an option. The purpose of such monitoring is to confirm abstinence, to detect body packers or to diagnose poisoning. Where confirmation of smoked cocaine (crack) is required the pyrolytic product methyl econidine or its nor-metabolite may be sought in urine.

Heroin

Clinical use

IMPORTANT FACTS

- Legally available for management of specified 'street' heroin users
- Opiate analgesic
- Heroin is typically injected, may be smoked or administered sub-cutaneously

Morphine is the active principal plasma metabolite, and the detection of morphine and metabolites has been the mainstay of urine monitoring for adherance to abuse withdrawal schemes. However the advent of the 'poppy seed defence' (natural sources of morphine in certain foodstuffs) means that detection of the heroin specific metabolite 6-monoacetyl morphine in urine is taken as conclusive proof, though it has a short plasma half-life. This metabolite is also detectable in oral fluid.

Structures of some drugs of abuse

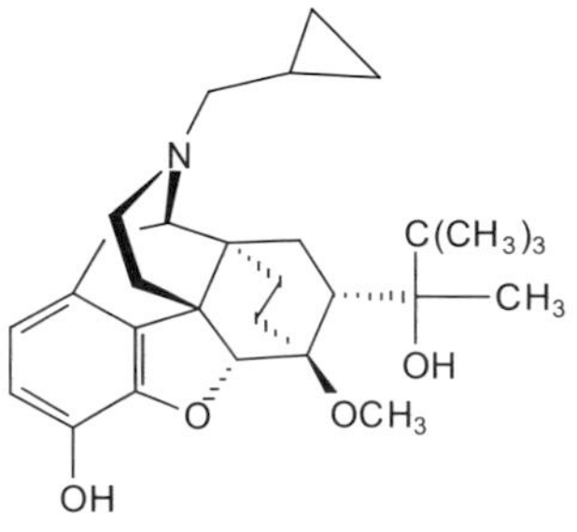

Buprenorphine

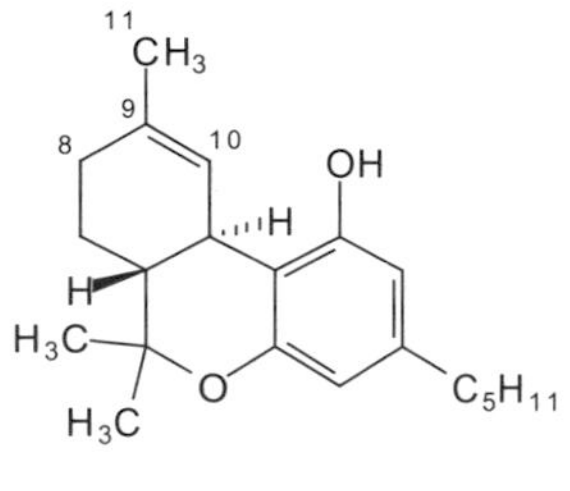

Δ^9-THC

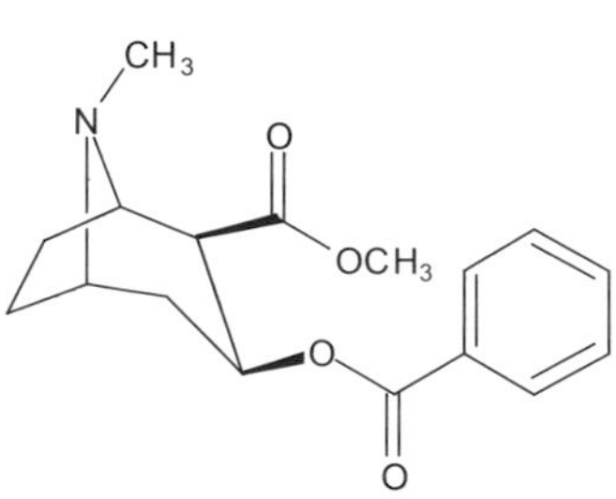

Cocaine

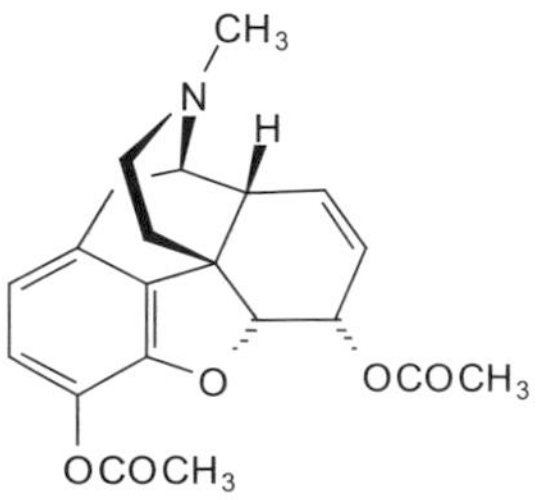

3,6-Diacetylmorphine
(Diamorphine, heroin)

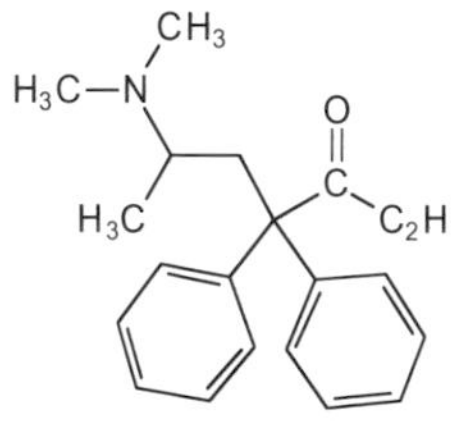

Methadone

IMMUNOSUPPRESSIVE DRUGS

Ciclosporin

Clinical use

IMPORTANT FACTS

Transplantation

- Organ transplantation – Prevention of graft rejection following kidney, liver, heart, combined heart-lung, lung or pancreas transplants. Treatment of transplant rejection in patients previously receiving other immunosuppressive agents
- Bone marrow transplantation – Prevention of graft rejection following bone marrow transplantation and prophylaxis of graft-versus-host disease (GVHD). Treatment of established graft-versus-host disease

Non-transplantation indications

- Psoriasis – Used in patients with severe psoriasis in whom conventional therapy is ineffective or inappropriate
- Atopic dermatitis – Short term treatment (8 weeks) of patients with severe atopic dermatitis in whom conventional therapy is ineffective or inappropriate
- Rheumatoid arthritis – Treatment of severe, active rheumatoid arthritis in patients in whom classical, slow-acting antirheumatic agents are inappropriate or ineffective
- Nephrotic syndrome – Treatment of steroid dependent or steroid resistant nephrotic syndrome (associated with adverse prognostic features) due to minimal change glomerulonephritis, focal segmental glomerulosclerosis or membranous glomerulonephritis in both adults and children
- Ulcerative colitis – Used in the treatment of refractory ulcerative colitis but this is an unlicensed indication

Ciclosporin (Neoral®, Novartis Pharmaceuticals UK Ltd) is a cyclic undecapeptide that was isolated from *Tolypocladium inflatum Gams* which in turn was isolated from soil samples collected from Wisconsin, USA and from the Hardanger Vidda fjord in Norway. One of the 11 amino acids, MeBmt (methylated (4R)-4-[(E)-2-butenyl]-4-methyl-L-threonine), is unique to ciclosporin. The drug was the first of a new class of immunosuppressant drugs, the calcineurin enzyme inhibitors.

Inhibition of this enzyme leads to inhibition of cytokine production and limits T-cell activation (tacrolimus has a similar mode of action). Ciclosporin is available for oral use as a solution and a capsule formulation; an intravenous preparation is also available.

Oral doses following transplantation are between 10 and 15 mg/kg/d for 1 to 2 weeks post-operatively then reduced gradually to 2 to 6 mg/kg/d for maintenance (dose is usually guided by blood ciclosporin concentration and renal function), in two divided doses.

In dermatology ciclosporin is initially given at 2.5 mg/kg/d in two divided doses and this may be increased to 5 mg/kg/d if response is not achieved. When used in dermatology the dose is usually guided by response to therapy and renal function, and treatment may be discontinued once a satisfactory response has been achieved although some patients may require continuous maintenance therapy. When used to treat nephrotic syndrome ciclosporin is initially given at 5 mg/kg/d, in two divided doses. The dose can then be slowly reduced according to efficacy, as measured by the degree of proteinuria and renal function, serum creatinine, to the lowest effective level.

The use of ciclosporin for the treatment of ulcerative colitis is unlicensed. Nevertheless, the drug is given to treat this condition by intravenous infusion of 2 mg/kg/d or oral drug administration. The dose can be adjusted by blood ciclosporin concentration and patient response. The drug also has several uses in veterinary medicine. Small changes in ciclosporin dose can result in either loss of efficacy or serious adverse effects. For this reason it is important that patients are maintained on the same formulation so ciclosporin should be prescribed by the proprietary brand name and not generically. The British National Formulary warns that *"because of differences in bioavailability, the brand of ciclosporin to be dispensed should be specified by the prescriber"*.

Pharmacokinetics

IMPORTANT FACTS

- Metabolised by the CYP3A enzyme system in the liver and the gut
- Substrate for the P-glycoprotein transporter system
- Metabolism is affected by genetic polymorphism of CYP3A4/CYP3A5 enzymes, but the clinical importance of this is unclear
- There are many clinically significant pharmacokinetic drug interactions

The pharmacokinetics of ciclosporin vary widely, both within-patient and between-patient. This variability, combined with a narrow therapeutic index, is the underlying rationale for therapeutic drug monitoring.

Ciclosporin is highly lipophilic and distributes extensively into body tissues including adipose tissue and liver. The drug's accumulation in red blood cells leads to an approximately 3-fold higher concentration in red cells compared with plasma. Within plasma the drug is extensively bound to plasma proteins, in excess of 98%. Ciclosporin is bound primarily to lipoproteins, including high-density, low-density and very-low-density lipoprotein, and, to a lesser extent, albumin. Although there is some evidence to suggest that the unbound concentration of the drug has a closer association with organ rejection than the total concentration, the measurement of unbound drug concentration is complex and cannot be performed easily in a clinical setting.

Oral bioavailability is low, about 38%, and varies between 20 and 60%. The low bioavailability is, in part, attributable to two major barriers to uptake in the gut wall, the efflux protein P-glycoprotein and the drug metabolising enzyme CYP3A. The genetic polymorphisms in the genes encoding for these enzymes account for much of the variability in absorption. However, unlike tacrolimus, for which clinically important variation has been shown, the clinical impact of these genetic polymorphisms is unclear. Ciclosporin is metabolised extensively, but there are no data to suggest that the metabolites exert any clinically significant pharmacological activity. In renal transplant patients the mode for CL/F is 6.3 mL/min/kg and for V_d is 6.4 L/kg. This equates to a half-life in blood of around 11.6 hours. However, in other patient studies the half-life of ciclosporin has been reported to be between 4.3 and 53.4 hours. In part this may reflect the many different methods used to measure ciclosporin in blood and plasma and the lack of standardisation and agreement between these analytical methods. Pharmacokinetic drug interactions are well documented, and mostly involve induction or inhibition of the CYP3A enzyme system or the P-glycoprotein efflux protein. In addition, interactions with foods or herbs that can influence these systems, such as grapefruit juice and St John's wort may occur.

In mycophenolate treated organ transplant recipients, lower mycophenolate plasma concentrations have been found in ciclosporin treated patients compared with those receiving tacrolimus. This interaction has been attributed to the reduction of the biliary excretion of mycophenolate glucuronide caused by ciclosporin inhibiting the MRP2 transporter system in the liver.

When ciclosporin, as Neoral®, is coadministered with sirolimus the blood concentrations of the latter drug increase 3.3-fold due to a pharmacokinetic interaction. However, the degree of increase appears to be formulation specific. When ciclosporin, as Gengraf®, is coadministered with sirolimus the increase in sirolimus C_{max} and AUC is smaller and sirolimus given with Gengraf® could not be considered to be bioequivalent to sirolimus given with Neoral®. A similar, interaction exists between everolimus and ciclosporin. Again there is a formulation specific interaction with everolimus; the AUC increase with Neoral® coadministration being significantly greater than the AUC increase with Sandimmune®.

SUMMARY OF CICLOSPORIN PHARMACOKINETICS (NEORAL®)

Parameter	Ciclosporin
Oral bioavailability (F)	0.38
Fraction excreted renally	<0.01
Fraction bound to plasma proteins	> 0.98
Clearance (corrected for bioavailability) (mL/min/kg)	6.3
Volume of distribution V_d (L/kg)	6.4
Elimination half-life (h)	11.6
Time to maximum concentration (h)	1.5

Toxicity

IMPORTANT FACTS

- Renal dysfunction is a serious adverse effect of ciclosporin
- Ciclosporin also causes raised blood pressure and hyperlipidaemia
- Adverse cosmetic effects (gingival hyperplasia and hypertrichosis) reduce quality of life
- Over immunosuppression is associated with infection and neoplasia

One reason to monitor ciclosporin is to avoid adverse effects. Whilst there is a wide overlap between the blood ciclosporin concentrations associated with unwanted effects and efficacy, the incidence of unwanted effects is concentration related and rises substantially at higher concentrations. Renal dysfunction is associated with the renal vasoconstrictive effect of ciclosporin and leads to chronic graft dysfunction. The adverse effects are minimised by maintaining exposure to the drug to the lowest consistent with efficacy and by the use of combined therapy with other drugs, such as mycophenolic acid or sirolimus, allowing dose minimisation of all drugs.

Monitoring therapy

IMPORTANT FACTS

- The concentration in blood is a better guide to effect than dose
- The recommended sample matrix is EDTA anticoagulated whole blood
- The recommended sampling times are C_0 (trough) or C_2 (2 hours post-dose)
- Target concentration ranges vary with time after transplantation, transplant type, concomitant drug therapy and analytical methods

Despite the imprecise relationship between blood ciclosporin concentration and the pharmacological effects of the drug, measurement of the drug concentration in blood is a better guide to therapy than knowledge of the dose administered.

The recommended sample matrix is whole blood because plasma concentrations vary considerably due to the temperature related variation in the distribution of the drug between red cells and plasma. EDTA is the recommended anticoagulant since heparin can be deactivated by haemolysis and EDTA causes fewer problems when samples are frozen and thawed prior to analysis.

Most laboratories use an immunoassay to monitor ciclosporin. Currently, there are at least seven in common use and they are based on a variety of techniques and run on several different analyser platforms. HPLC with mass-spectrometric detection is now the method of choice in around 8% of laboratories worldwide. This proportion of laboratories is increasing as this technique has some advantages, due to the absence of interference from metabolites of the drug and increased sensitivity compared with the immunoassays. On average, immunoassay results are about 10-15% higher than those produced by chromatographic techniques. However, the difference can be much larger in the setting of liver dysfunction, leading to a higher proportion of ciclosporin metabolites which cross-react with the antibodies used in the immunoassay kits.

The ciclosporin concentration in blood samples is stable for more than one week at ambient temperatures of 20-25°C and for at least a year at -20°C. Thus, samples can be shipped to central laboratories without cooling, although it is good practice to store samples refrigerated at 4°C prior to analysis.

Target blood concentration ranges based on the use of a C_0 measurement vary with concomitant therapy, the transplant type, time after transplantation and the analytical method used. Following kidney transplantation, a typical target concentration is 200 to 400 µg/L in the month following transplantation when ciclosporin is used with corticosteroids and mycophenate. Target concentrations in stable patients are of the order 100 to 150 µg/L. The target ranges used in different transplant units can vary considerably despite using the same immuno-suppressant regimen. This is, at least in part, because the C_0 concentration ranges have been arrived at empirically by clinical 'experience' and 'judgement' and have not been prospectively tested for outcome.

The use of ciclosporin concentrations two hours post dose, C_2, to monitor therapy has theoretical advantages over C_0 measurements in that C_2 is predictive of expo-sure while C_0 is not. C_2 measurements have been shown to closely correlate with both efficacy and toxicity whereas the data relating C_0 concentrations to clinical events is equivocal. Several clinical trials in transplantation have shown stronger association between C_2 and outcome than C_0. In addition, C_2 concentrations have been tested prospectively in a concentration controlled clinical trial in *de novo* kidney transplantation. The target C_2 concentration immediately following trans-plantation is 1500 µg/L and this is tapered over the next six months to 700 µg/L.

Currently, there are no generic formulations of ciclosporin on the market in the UK. However, there are concerns that the introduction of multiple formulations of ciclosporin will be deleterious to patient care. Despite these new formulations needing to meet current bioequivalence standards these may not be sufficiently stringent to ensure therapeutic equivalence in patients and there is some evidence that this may indeed be the case. The other issue is that although a formulation may deliver the same average bioavailability as existing formulations individual patients may not absorb the same amount of ciclosporin from each formulation. Thus 'generic' prescribing or unplanned switching from one brand to another could result in significant under or over dosing and hence therapeutic failure or toxicity. Due to differences in individual bioavailability between different oral formulations of ciclosporin, it is important that medical practitioners, pharma-cists, and patients are aware that substitution between formulations should only be done with appropriate monitoring of ciclosporin blood concentrations, serum creatinine concentrations and blood pressure. Current recommendations are that ciclosporin should be prescribed by brand and that if a patient is to be switched from one brand to another then this should be carried out in a specialist centre where the patient can receive appropriate, expert, monitoring.

As for all immunosuppressive drug measurements, the interpretation of a blood ciclosporin concentration must be made with regard to such factors as: the method used to measure the drug, the time interval between the sample and the last dose, the clinical indication for the use of the drug, the duration of therapy and other drug therapy. The unthinking use of 'therapeutic ranges' should be discouraged.

Mycophenolate

Clinical use

IMPORTANT FACTS

- Licensed to prevent rejection in kidney, heart and liver transplant patients, in combination with ciclosporin and corticosteroids
- Also widely used in combination with tacrolimus, sirolimus and everolimus
- Occasionally used in a stand-alone regimen for the prevention of rejection in patients at low immunological risk

There are two formulations. CellCept® (Roche) is a pro-drug – mycophenolate mofetil (MMF) – which is hydrolysed rapidly following oral administration to form the active drug mycophenolic acid (MPA). Most data relating to monitoring of this drug refer to this formulation. Myfortic® (Novartis Pharmaceuticals) is the enteric coated sodium salt of MPA (EC-MPS). The molecular weights of the two formulations differ, so that 1 g MMF is equivalent to 720 mg EC-MPS. Using these relative doses the two formulations are bioequivalent.

MMF is available as 250 mg capsules and 500 mg tablets. Following kidney transplantation the recommended starting dose is 1g twice daily. Following heart and liver transplantation the recommended starting dose is 1.5 g twice daily. An intravenous formulation is also available. EC-MPS is available as 180 mg and 360 mg tablets. It is licensed following kidney transplantation with a starting dose of 720 mg twice daily.

MPA is a reversible, non-competitive, inhibitor of the enzyme inosine monophosphate dehydrogenase (IMPDH), a key enzyme in the *de novo* synthesis of purines. Inhibition of this enzyme blocks lymphocyte proliferation. Depletion of guanosine nucleotides via the action of MPA influences both DNA synthesis and glycosylation of adhesion molecules. As a result, MPA blocks proliferation of T and B lymphocytes and inhibits antibody production.

Pharmacokinetics

Important Facts

- Rapidly absorbed from the MMF formulation
- Prolonged absorption from EC-MPS formulation
- Highly bound to plasma proteins, principally albumin
- Principal metabolite is a phenolic glucuronide (MPAG)
- MPA and MPAG are renally excreted
- Clinically significant pharmacokinetic interaction with ciclosporin

Following oral administration of MMF the ester is hydrolysed very rapidly to give MPA and hydroxyethyl morpholine. MMF is, essentially, undetectable after oral dosing. Following intravenous administration the plasma half-life of MMF is less than two minutes.

MPA reaches its maximum concentration very rapidly following ingestion of the MMF formulation. The pharmacokinetic difference between MMF and EC-MPA is that the latter has to pass through the stomach before absorption of MPA starts. As a result, peak concentrations are generally delayed beyond two hours after dosing. However, if the formulation is taken with food, and there is delayed gastric emptying, then the time to maximum concentration may be delayed by more than five hours. MPA is extensively bound to plasma proteins, mostly to albumin, but the free-fraction in plasma varies. It can be as little as 1% but increases up to about 7% if albumin concentrations are low or if patients suffer renal dysfunction. Since it is the free-fraction that exerts pharmacological activity, measurement of total MPA concentrations in plasma may not reflect the concentration of active drug.

The principal metabolite is formed by conjugation in the liver, to produce the phenolic glucuronide (MPAG). This compound is excreted in urine and is not pharmacologically active. However, its kinetics are complicated by enterohepatic recycling. Following excretion into bile, MPAG deglucuronidation occurs in the intestine, followed by re-absorption of MPA. This phenomenon may be apparent when the MPA plasma concentration profile is measured over a full dose interval, as a distinct second absorption peak may occur at about 6-8 hours after ingestion. The concentrations of MPAG may exceed those of MPA several fold (20 to 100 times more) particularly so in patients with poor renal function.

In addition to MPAG a phenolic glucoside and an acyl glucuronide have also been identified. *In vitro*, the acyl glucuronide has been shown to have pharmacological activity and has been implicated in some of the adverse effects of MPA.

Clearance of MPA is time-dependent, decreasing over the first few weeks following transplantation, probably in association with changes in plasma albumin concentration and renal function. As a result, MPA exposure increases per unit dose over the first three months after transplantation.

An important pharmacokinetic drug interaction is that between ciclosporin and MPA, leading to a significant reduction in MPA exposure when the drugs are co-administered. This interaction appears to be caused by a ciclosporin-related reduction in biliary excretion of MPAG. The underlying mechanism is inhibition of the anion transporter, multidrug resistance-associated protein 2 (MRP2), found in the bile canilicular membrane of hepatocytes. A reduction in MPAG entering the gut in bile leads to a reduction in the enterohepatic recycling of MPA.

There is the potential for pharmacokinetic drug interactions between MPA and other drugs that are metabolised by uridine diphosphate-glucuronosyltransferase isoenzymes and those that interact with the MRP2 transporter system. Recently, a reduction in MPA exposure was noted in patients co-prescribed rifampicin. The underlying mechanism was thought to be induction of glucuronidation by rifampicin, together with associated alterations in MRP2 transport of MPAG into the gut.

Finally, the unbound concentration of MPA can be increased by drugs that have a high affinity for albumin binding sites, by high concentrations of MPAG, and by uraemia.

SUMMARY OF MYCOPHENOLATE PHARMACOKINETICS (MMF FORMULATION)

Parameter	MMF
Oral bioavailability (F)	0.95
Fraction excreted renally	>0.90
Fraction bound to plasma proteins	0.98
Clearance (corrected for bioavailability) (mL/min/kg)	Varies (see text)
Volume of distribution V_d (L/kg)	1.6
Elimination half-life (h)	17
Time to maximum concentration (h)	1.0

Toxicity

IMPORTANT FACTS

- Gastrointestinal adverse effects are common
- Therapy with MPA is associated with an increased incidence of haematological adverse effects
- Over-immunosuppression is associated with infection and neoplasia

The drug is generally well tolerated. The most frequently recorded adverse effects are those affecting the gastrointestinal system, including nausea, vomiting, diarrhoea and abdominal pain. The acyl glucuronide has been implicated in the aetiology of these effects, secondary to its pro-inflammatory actions. The enteric coated formulation was developed with the aim of reducing the gastrointestinal adverse effects associated with MMF, by targeting the release of MPA in the small intestine.

There is an increased incidence of leucopenia, anaemia and thrombocytopenia in patients receiving MPA, and the incidence of opportunistic infections is raised.

In general, adverse effects have tended to correlate with dose, rather than MPA concentrations, although some centres have reported an association between MPA concentrations and adverse events. It should be remembered that many of the adverse effects noted for MPA could have multiple causes, so it is not surprising that determining a clear relationship with MPA concentration has proved elusive. Suffice to note that adverse effects leading to dose reduction or discontinuation of MPA are associated with an increased risk of poor long-term outcome.

Monitoring therapy

IMPORTANT FACTS

- Within-patient variability for pre-dose concentrations is high
- The recommended sample matrix is EDTA anticoagulated plasma or serum
- There are well defined limited sampling algorithms to estimate AUC
- Most data on monitoring relate to the MMF formulation

Measurement of MPA is relatively easy. Plasma is the matrix of choice and concentrations are much higher than those associated with the calcineurin inhibitors or the mTOR binding drugs; pre-dose concentrations are of the order 1-3 mg/L in plasma. The drug is usually measured by high-performance liquid chromatography (HPLC) with either ultraviolet or mass-spectrometric detection, or by an immunoassay based on the enzyme-multiplied immunoassay technique (EMIT). There is a bias between the measurements obtained by these two techniques, attributed to antibody cross-reactivity with the acyl glucuronide. Typically, immunoassay results are about 20% higher than those produced by HPLC. In addition, it should be noted that the immunoassay cross-reacts with MMF, so is not suitable for the measurement of MPA in samples collected during or shortly after intravenous therapy with MMF. There is an enzyme receptor assay in development, based on inhibition of IMPDH. Preliminary data show good agreement between this assay and HPLC.

The pre-dose (trough) concentration shows substantial within-patient variability, with a coefficient of variation, for the MMF formulation, of about 50%. Thus, isolated measurements made pre-dose should be interpreted with caution. For the EC-MPS formulation the situation is complicated by the possibility of delayed gastric emptying, resulting in apparently high pre-dose concentrations. The impact of this effect is to give rise to pre-dose concentrations of the order 8-12 mg/L in a minority of measurements. It is arguable whether the use of pre-dose measurements is useful for patients receiving EC-MPS, except for adherence purposes and, in any event, careful note must be made of which formulation has been used before interpretation of a pre-dose concentrations can be made.

Because pre-dose concentrations vary so widely, and are poor reflections of total MPA exposure, efforts have been made to develop simple sampling strategies to calculate area under the time/concentration curve (AUC). There are substantial data to show that efficacy is related to exposure, as measured by AUC, based on a large, multicentre, randomised concentration-controlled trial (RCCT) in kidney transplant patients, and from a number of single centre studies. The RCCT used an algorithm based on collecting five timed samples during the first two hours after dosing. It was noted that efficacy, in association with ciclosporin, was associated with exposures in excess of 30 mg/h/L. Subsequently, other groups have developed algorithms based on fewer samples, usually three in the first two hours post-dose, to calculate AUC. These algorithms follow the kinetics of the MMF formulation and cannot be used for the EC-MPS formulation. It is possible to estimate AUC for EC-MPS, but samples must be collected up to about 6-8 hours post-dose to obtain a good estimate.

There have been some attempts to measure the pharmacodynamics of MPA by measuring the activity of IMPDH in blood. The methodology is complex and work has been confined to specialist centres. The data show that activity of this enzyme is, intrinsically, highly variable and that this variability may contribute to between-patient differences in efficacy.

It can be useful to measure the concentration of MPAG in plasma although, of course, a chromatographic technique is required. High concentrations of MPAG displace MPA from its plasma protein binding sites, increasing the free-fraction of the drug. Research on the implications of the acyl glucuronide metabolite is hampered by its lack of availability as a commercial product.

The consensus is that MPA kinetics are highly variable and that knowledge of the dose alone is a poor reflection of exposure. Some measure of exposure, preferably AUC, is probably helpful in the early period following transplantation, to ensure that adequate exposure has been achieved. An AUC in the range 30-60 mg*h/L is recommended, and this holds true whichever MPA formulation is used. If it is not possible to make an AUC measurement then pre-dose concentrations may be useful, but a series of two or three should be measured to take into account the wide variability of this parameter. Concentrations of about 1-2 mg/L are recommended following kidney transplantation and about 1-3 mg/L following heart transplantation. One should also consider that MPA is usually only one part of the immunosuppressive drug regimen and that measurement of other drugs, such as ciclosporin and tacrolimus, should not be forgotten.

As for all immunosuppressive drug measurements, the interpretation of an MPA plasma concentration must be made with regard to such factors as: the method used to measure the drug, the clinical indication for the use of the drug, the time interval between the sample and the last dose, the duration of therapy and other drug therapy. Because there is a substantial body of data on the measurement of AUC, some thought should be given to the use of limited sample strategies to estimate this parameter. The unthinking use of 'therapeutic ranges' should be discouraged.

Sirolimus

Clinical use

IMPORTANT FACTS

- Licensed for use in kidney transplant patients at low to moderate risk of rejection
- Normally used in combination with a calcineurin inhibitor and corticosteroids for 2 to 3 months following transplantation
- Licensed for prolonged use with corticosteroids only if use of the calcineurin inhibitor can be progressively discontinued

Sirolimus (Rapamune®, Wyeth Pharmaceuticals) is a macrocyclic lactone derived from the actinomycete *Streptomyces hygroscopicus*. It was originally isolated from soil samples collected from Rapa Nui (Easter Island). Although structurally related to tacrolimus, sirolimus has a different mode of action. Both drugs bind to a binding protein, FK binding protein (FKBP-12), but sirolimus then binds to a protein kinase – mammalian target of rapamycin (mTOR). Binding of the sirolimus-FKBP complex to mTOR blocks signal transduction in the second phase of T-cell activation, resulting in the blockade of interleukin-2 induced T-cell proliferation.

Sirolimus is a potent immunosuppressive drug, available in two oral formulations, a liquid and tablet. Most pharmacokinetic data relate to the liquid formulation. Although absorption from the tablet formulation tends to be slightly higher than from the liquid formulation, the two formulations have therapeutic equivalence at a dose of 2 mg daily. Following a loading dose of 6 mg the usual starting dose is 2 mg per day, with subsequent dose adjustments made on the basis of blood concentration measurements. Since being licensed for use in kidney transplantation, in association with ciclosporin, a number of sirolimus protocols have been investigated and the drug has been used for other transplant indications. Attention has focused on combining sirolimus with tacrolimus and/or mycophenolate, in heart, liver and pancreas transplantation.

Pharmacokinetics

IMPORTANT FACTS

- Metabolised by CYP3A in the liver and the gut
- Substrate for the P-glycoprotein transporter system
- Many clinically significant pharmacokinetic drug interactions
- Comparatively long plasma half-life

Sirolimus is absorbed rapidly via the oral route. It has a relatively low bioavailability, less than 15%, which can be influenced by concomitant medication. When co-administered with the microemulsion formulation of ciclosporin the absorption of sirolimus is enhanced, almost doubling the effective dose. For this reason the recommendation is to give sirolimus 4 hours after dosing ciclosporin, but this advice is often ignored, and the dose of sirolimus adjusted based on therapeutic drug monitoring. However, this interaction should be remembered if ciclosporin is withdrawn from therapy as, to maintain adequate exposure, an increase in sirolimus dose can be anticipated. Sirolimus is extensively distributed into body tissues, with a particularly high uptake by red blood cells. The blood:plasma ratio is in excess of 30 and only about 2.5% of sirolimus in plasma is unbound.

Sirolimus is extensively metabolised to monohydroxy-, dihydroxy-, demethyl- and didemethyl-metabolites. Whilst unchanged sirolimus represents less than half the sirolimus-derived compounds in the bloodstream, there is no evidence that the metabolites contribute significantly to the clinical efficacy of the drug. Hence, measurement of individual metabolites as a guide to therapy is not necessary.

Because sirolimus is a substrate for both the CYP3A and P-glycoprotein a broad range of interactions with other drugs and dietary components have been identified, in line with those noted for ciclosporin and tacrolimus. Although ciclosporin impacts on sirolimus kinetics, there is no evidence that the reverse is the case, but one study has suggested that sirolimus lowers exposure to tacrolimus. There is evidence that, as for tacrolimus, patients who are producers of the CYP3A5 enzyme metabolise sirolimus faster than those without this enzyme. Thus, patients who are CYP3A5 producers will require higher doses of sirolimus and may take longer to reach target concentrations.

Negligible amounts of sirolimus are excreted in urine. Elimination of the drug is via the liver into bile, clearance approximating to liver blood flow. Dose reductions should be made in patients who develop cholestasis. Sirolimus has a relatively long plasma half-life of about 60 hours. Thus, it is common practice to use a loading dose at the start of therapy, and it takes over a week to achieve steady state after a dose alteration.

SUMMARY OF SIROLIMUS PHARMACOKINETICS
Toxicity

Parameter	Sirolimus
Oral bioavailability (F)*	0.14
Fraction excreted renally	< 0.01
Fraction bound to plasma proteins	0.92
Clearance (corrected for bioavailability) (mL/min/kg)	2.8
Volume of distribution V_d (L/kg)	12.0
Elimination half-life (h)	62
Time to maximum concentration (h)	1 - 2
*except when co-administered with ciclosporin (see text)	

IMPORTANT FACTS

- Use of sirolimus is associated with:
  - anaemia, leucopenia and thrombocytopenia
  - hypertriglyceridaemia and hypercholesterolaemia
  - lymphocele formation and impaired wound healing
- Prolonged use of sirolimus and calcineurin inhibitors is associated with a synergistic effect on nephrotoxicity

The haematological effects and the impact on lipid indices are related to sirolimus concentrations in blood. They are usually managed by dose reduction and the use of lipid lowering therapy. The lipid abnormalities are not associated with an excess of cardiovascular disease in sirolimus treated patients compared with those receiving long-term calcineurin inhibitor therapy.

There has been particular interest in the use of sirolimus because it is, intrinsically, not nephrotoxic. This characteristic has led to clinical studies that have focused on the possibility of reducing, or eliminating, ciclosporin from the immunosuppressive regimen, to reduce the incidence of calcineurin-related renal damage. The pivotal studies compared full dose ciclosporin therapy with the addition of sirolimus, followed by randomisation to continuation with this regimen or ciclosporin elimination after three months. Clinically, the results were comparable in each arm of the study, but renal function improved in the patients withdrawn from ciclosporin. This improvement was still evident beyond two years after transplantation. However, with increasing use of the drug, in combination with either ciclosporin or tacrolimus, enhanced calcineurin-related nephrotoxicity has been observed. This has resulted in poorer long-term graft survival in kidney transplant patients remaining on the combination of sirolimus and a calcineurin inhibitor. It has been suggested that the inhibitory effect of sirolimus on P-glyco-protein activity could result in reduced efflux of ciclosporin from kidney cells in those patients receiving combined therapy with the two drugs.

The incidence of infection in sirolimus treated patients is similar to that noted in patients receiving other immunosuppressive drugs. There is a trend for sirolimus treated patients to record a lower incidence of post-transplant malignancies.

Monitoring therapy

IMPORTANT FACTS

- The concentration in blood is a better guide to effect than dose
- The recommended sample matrix is EDTA anticoagulated whole blood
- The recommended sampling time is C_0 (trough)
- Target concentration ranges are dependent on the analytical method

The relationship between sirolimus concentrations in blood and efficacy/toxicity was studied intensively during the early clinical evaluation of this drug. Data were collected from concentration-controlled studies which were then used to establish validated reference concentration ranges as a guide to dose adjustment. There is a good correlation between exposure, as measured by the area under the time-concentration curve (AUC) and the sirolimus pre-dose concentration in blood. Sirolimus has a relatively long half-life so is given only once daily, unlike ciclosporin and tacrolimus which are usually given twice daily. The target concentration ranges derived from the pivotal studies were based on the use of sirolimus combined with ciclosporin. Target concentrations for the use of sirolimus with other drug combinations are being developed.

A large proportion of laboratories measure sirolimus using high-performance liquid chromatography (HPLC), with either ultraviolet (UV) or mass-spectrometric (MS) detection. An immunoassay, currently based on the Abbott IMx platform, is widely available. Immunoassay results are about 20-30% higher than those produced by HPLC methods. Care should be taken when using published target ranges to ensure that they are appropriate for the analytical method being used.

Therapeutic drug monitoring of sirolimus is a regulatory requirement, and is particularly advised when patients suffer hepatic impairment, if CYP3A enzyme inducers or inhibitors are given concurrently, and if ciclosporin dose is changed. When ciclosporin is prescribed with sirolimus there must be a consistent time interval between taking each drug to minimise variability of the concentration of sirolimus. When given with ciclosporin, during the three months following transplantation, the target range for sirolimus blood concentrations is 4 - 12 µg/L using a chromatographic assay. The recommendation is to increase this range to 12 - 20 µg/L when ciclosporin is discontinued, although some centres use lower ranges for long-term therapy depending upon the concomitant therapy used.

Because such a high proportion of sirolimus in blood is concentrated in the red cell, it is essential that blood samples are mixed thoroughly prior to analysis. Adequate mixing ensures that underestimation of the sirolimus concentration, due to red cells settling in the blood tube, is avoided.

As for all immunosuppressive drug measurements, the interpretation of a sirolimus blood concentration must be made with regard to such factors as: the method used to measure the drug, the clinical indication for the use of the drug, the duration of therapy and other drug therapy. The time interval between the sample and the last dose must also be taken into account but, since the drug has a long half-life, the 24 hour pre-dose sample tends to be relatively unaffected by fluctuations in the time of dosing. The unthinking use of 'therapeutic ranges' should be discouraged.

Note on everolimus

Everolimus is an analogue of sirolimus (40-o-(2-hydroxyethyl) rapamycin). The chemical modification results in everolimus being more polar than sirolimus. The plasma half-life of everolimus is about 30 hours and the volume of distribution is markedly lower. The drug is not licensed for use in the UK or the Irish Republic, but is licensed for use in many European countries. Monitoring of the drug is recommended and two methods are commonly used to measure the drug, HPLC/MS and an immunoassay produced by Seradyn. Concentrations in blood associated with efficacy are of the order 3 - 8 µg/L.

Tacrolimus

Clinical use

IMPORTANT FACTS

- Licensed to prevent rejection following kidney, liver and heart allograft transplantation
- Licensed for the treatment of allograft rejection in patients resistant to treatment with other immunosuppressives
- Used to prevent rejection in other transplant indications, e.g. lung and intestine
- Used in the treatment of some autoimmune diseases

Tacrolimus (Prograf®, Astellas) is an immunosuppressive drug that is an inhibitor of calcineurin. For use following transplantation it is available as a capsule formulation and as an intravenous preparation. Oral doses following kidney transplantation are of the order 0.1 - 0.2 mg/kg/day, in two divided doses. Dose adjustments are normally guided by TDM.

In addition to its use in solid organ transplant rejection, tacrolimus is used in the treatment of some autoimmune diseases and in the treatment of atopic dermatitis. For the latter condition there is an ointment formulation (Protopic®). Monitoring of the drug in blood is not normally necessary when it is used to treat auto-immune diseases.

Pharmacokinetics

IMPORTANT FACTS

- Metabolised by CYP3A in the liver and the gut
- Substrate for the P-glycoprotein
- Metabolism significantly affected by genetic polymorphism of CYP3A4/CYP3A5 enzymes
- Many clinically significant pharmacokinetic drug interactions

The pharmacokinetics of tacrolimus vary widely, both within-patient and between-patient. This variability, combined with a narrow therapeutic index, is the underlying rationale for therapeutic drug monitoring.

Tacrolimus is highly lipophilic and distributes extensively into body tissues. Its accumulation in red blood cells leads to an approximately 20 - 30-fold higher concentration in red cells compared with plasma. Within plasma the drug is extensively bound to plasma proteins, in excess of 98%, mostly to α_1-acid glyco-protein and albumin.

Oral bioavailability is about 20%, but varies widely. The low bioavailability is, in part, attributable to two major barriers to uptake in the gut wall, P-glycoprotein and CYP3A. A genetic polymorphism in the gene encoding for the enzyme results in some subjects producing both CYP3A4 and CYP3A5, both of which metabolise tacrolimus. There are ethnic differences in the expression of CYP3A5; it is expressed by about 80% of Blacks compared with only 15% of Caucasians. As a result, CYP3A5 expressors require higher doses of the drug compared with non-expressors.

Tacrolimus is metabolised extensively, but there are no data to suggest that the metabolites exert significant pharmacological activity. Tacrolimus is a low clear-ance drug, the major route of elimination being bile. Reduction in liver function can lead to prolonged elimination and a build-up of tacrolimus metabolites in the blood. Following kidney transplantation, increased oral bioavailability of tacrolimus has been noted in patients with severe diarrhoea. The likely mechanism for this effect is a decrease in the activity of intestinal P-glycoprotein activity. Pharmacokinetic drug interactions are well documented and, mostly, involve induction or inhibition of CYP3A or P-glycoprotein. In addition, possible interactions with foods or herbs that can influence these systems, such as grapefruit juice and St John's wort, should be remembered.

SUMMARY OF TACROLIMUS PHARMACOKINETICS

Parameter	Tacrolimus
Oral bioavailability (F)	0.20 - 0.23
Fraction excreted renally	< 0.01
Fraction bound to plasma proteins	> 0.98
Clearance (corrected for bioavailability) (mL/min/kg)	0.09
Volume of distribution V_d (L/kg)	0.5 - 1.4
Elimination half-life (h)	10 - 20
Time to maximum concentration (h)	1 - 3

Toxicity

IMPORTANT FACTS

- Renal dysfunction is a serious adverse effect
- Tacrolimus raises blood pressure
- New onset diabetes occurs in more than 10% of patients
- Over immunosuppression is associated with infection and neoplasia

Whilst there is a wide overlap between the blood tacrolimus concentrations associated with unwanted effects and efficacy, the incidence of unwanted effects rises substantially at higher blood concentration. Renal dysfunction is associated with the renal vasoconstrictive effect of tacrolimus and leads to chronic graft dysfunction. The adverse effects are minimised by maintaining exposure to the drug to the lowest consistent with efficacy and by the use of combined therapy with other drugs, such as mycophenolic acid or sirolimus, allowing dose minimisation of all drugs.

Monitoring therapy

IMPORTANT FACTS

- The concentration in blood is a better guide to therapeutic effect than dose
- The recommended sample matrix is EDTA anticoagulated whole blood
- The recommended sampling time is C_0 (trough)
- Target concentration ranges vary with transplant type and other drug therapy and method of analysis

Despite the imprecise relationship between blood tacrolimus concentration and the pharmacological effects of the drug, measurement of the drug is a better guide to prescription than knowledge of the dose administered. The recommended sample matrix is whole blood because plasma concentrations are below the measurable range of almost any assay technique available and there is a temperature related variation in the distribution of the drug between red cells and plasma. EDTA is the recommended anticoagulant since this causes fewer problems when samples are frozen and thawed prior to analysis.

Most laboratories use an immunoassay to monitor tacrolimus. Currently, two are in common use, based on MEIA (Abbott Diagnostics) or EMIT (Dade Behring) technology. There is a growing use of HPLC with mass-spectrometric detection and this technique has some advantages, due to the absence of interference from metabolites of the drug and increased sensitivity compared with the immunoassays. On average, immunoassay results are about 10 - 15% higher than those produced by chromatographic techniques. However, the difference can be much larger in the setting of liver dysfunction, leading to a higher proportion of tacrolimus metabolites which cross-react with the anti-tacrolimus antibodies. There is some evidence that the MEIA technique is influenced by low haematocrit.

Tacrolimus in blood samples is stable for more than one week at 20 - 25°C and for at least a year at -20°C. Thus, samples can be shipped to central laboratories without cooling, although it is good practice to store samples refrigerated at 4°C prior to analysis. Because the concentration in red cells is high compared with plasma, samples should be thoroughly mixed prior to analysis.

It is thought that the pre-dose (C_0) concentration is a good reflection of total exposure. Target concentration ranges are based on the use of a C_0 measurement and vary with concomitant therapy and the transplant indication. Following kidney transplantation, a typical target concentration is 15 µg/L, when the drug is used with corticosteroids and mycophenolic acid. Target concentrations in stable patients are of the order 5 - 10 µg/L.

A modified release formulation of tacrolimus is being tested. The data from clinical trials in stable transplant patients suggests that once daily dosing of the new formulation can be substituted for twice daily dosing of the original formulation, using equivalent doses of both formulations. The implications of switching formulations for target concentrations is not certain at this stage.

As for all immunosuppressive drug measurements, the interpretation of a blood tacrolimus concentration must be made with regard to such factors as: the method used to measure the drug, the time interval between the sample and the last dose, the clinical indication for the use of the drug, the duration of therapy and other drug therapy. The unthinking use of 'therapeutic ranges' should be discouraged.

Structures of some immunosuppressive drugs

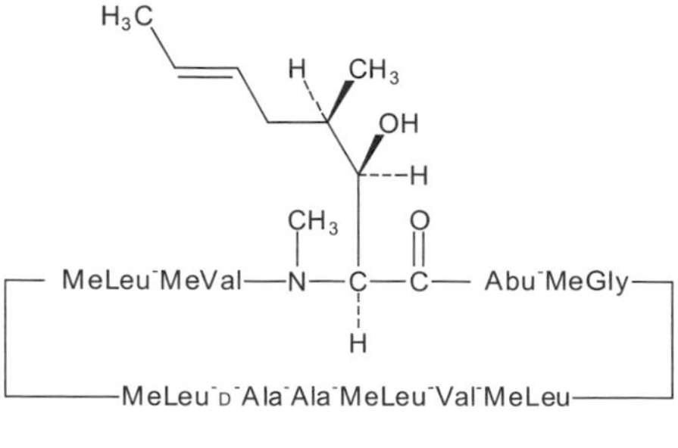

Cyclosporin A

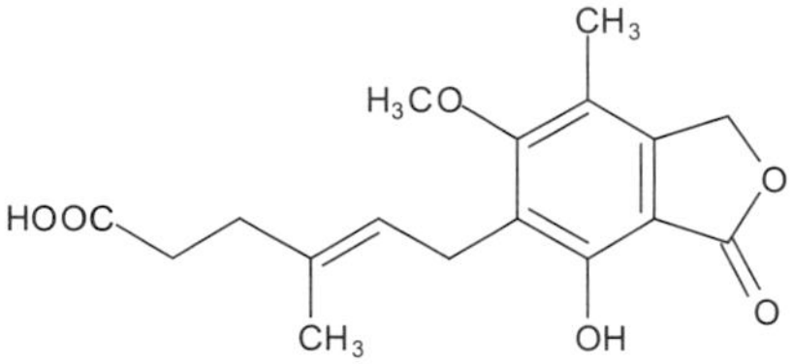

Mycophenolic acid

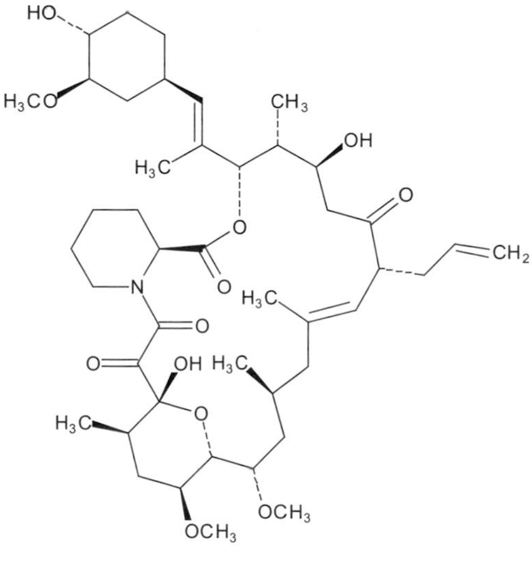

Tacrolimus

Further reading

Antibiotics

Aminoglycosides

Begg EJ, Barclay ML, Kirkpatrick CM. The therapeutic monitoring of antimicrobial agents. Br J Clin Pharmacol 2001; **52 Suppl 1:** 35S–43S

Nicolau DP, Freeman CD, Belliveau PP, Nightingale CH, Ross JW, Quintiliani R. Experience with a once-daily aminoglycoside program administered to 2,184 adult patients. Antimicrob Agents Chemother 1995; **29:** 650-655.

Touw DJ, Neef C, Thomson AH, Vinks AA. Cost-effectiveness of therapeutic drug monitoring – a systemic review. Ther Drug Monit 2005; **27:** 10-17

Glycopeptide antibiotics

McGowan AP. Pharmacodynamics, pharmacokinetics and therapeutic drug monitoring of glycopeptides.Ther Drug Monit 1998; **20:** 473-477.

Anti-cancer drugs

Methotrexate

Ackland SP, Schlisky RL. High-dose methotrexate: a critical reappraisal. J Clin Oncol 1987; **5:** 2017-2031.

Borchers AT, Keen CL, Cheema GS, Gershwin ME. The use of methotrexate in rheumatoid arthritis. Semin Arthritis Rheum 2004; **34:** 465-483.

Anti-convulsants

Bergin AM, Connolly M. New antiepileptic drug therapies. Neurol Clin 2002; 20: 1163-1182

Carbamazepine

Bertilsson L, Tomson T. Clinical pharmacokinetics and pharmacological effects of carbamazepine and carbamazepine 10,11-epoxide: an update. Clin Pharmacokinet 1986; **11:** 177-198.

Editorial. Carbamazepine update. Lancet 1989; **ii:** 595-597.

Ethosuximide

Goren MZ, Onat E. Ethosuximide: from bench to bedside. CNS Drug Rev 2007; **13:** 224-239.

Millership JS, Mifsud J, Galea D, McRoberts WC, Hamilton JT. Chiral aspects of the human metabolism of ethosuximide. Biopharm Drug Dispos 2005 **26:** 225-232.

Lamotrigine

Bialer M. Comparative pharmacokinetics of the newer antiepileptic drugs. Clin Pharmacokinet 1993; **24:** 441-452.

Brodie MJ. Lamotrigine. Lancet 1992; **339:** 1397-1400.

Oxcarbazepine

May TW, Korn-Merker E, Rambeck B. Clinical pharmacokinetics of oxcarbazepine. Clin Pharmacokinet 2003; 42: 1023-1042

Phenobarbital

Browne TR, Evans JE, Szabo GK, Evans BA, Greenblatt DJ. Studies with stable isotopes II: phenobarbital pharmacokinetics during monotherapy. J Clin Pharmacol 1985; **28:** 51-58

Eadie MJ, Heazlewood RL, Tyrer JH. How worthwhile is plasma primidone measurement? Clin Exp Neurol 1981; **18:** 123-131.

Phenytoin

Aronson JK, Hardman M, Reynolds DJM. ABC of monitoring drug therapy: phenytoin. BMJ 1992; **305:** 1215-1218.

Levine M, Chang T. Therapeutic drug monitoring of phenytoin: rationale and current status. Clin Pharmacokinet 1990; **19:** 341-358.

Richens A. Clinical pharmacokinetics of phenytoin. Clin Pharmacokinet 1979; **4:** 153-169.

Valproate

Chadwick DW. Concentration-effect relationships of valproic acid. Clin Pharmacokinet 1985; **10:** 155-163.

Schobben F, van der Kleijn E, Vree TB. Therapeutic monitoring of valproic acid. Ther Drug Monit 1980; **2:** 61-71.
Zaccara M, Messori A, Moroni F. Clinical pharmacokinetics of valproic acid – 1988. Clin Pharmacokinet 1988; **15:** 367-389.

Anti-depressants

Mitchell PB. Therapeutic drug monitoring of psychotropic medications. Br J Clin Pharmacol 2001; **52 Suppl 1:** 45S – 54S.

Standards of laboratory practice – antidepressant drug monitoring. National Academy of Clinical Biochemistry. Clin Chem 1998; **44:** 1073-1084

Antipsychotics

Flanagan RJ. Therapeutic drug monitoring of antipsychotic drugs. CPD Clinical Biochemistry 2006; **7:** 3-18.

Jann MW, Grimsley SR, Gray EC, Chang WH. Pharmacokinetics and pharmaco-dynamics of clozapine. Clin Pharmacokinet 1993; **24:** 161-176.

Kirchheiner J, Nickchen K, Bauer M, Wong ML, Licinio J, Roots I, *et al.* Pharmacogenetics of antidepressants and antipsychotics: the contribution of allelic variations to the phenotype of drug response. Mol Psychiatry 2004; **9:** 442-473.

Perel JM, Jann MW. Antipsychotics In: Applied Pharmacokinetics & Pharmacodynamics. Principles of Therapeutic Drug Monitoring 4th Edition. Eds Burton ME, Shaw LM, Schentag JJ, Evans WE. Lippincott Williams & Wilkins: Philadelphia. 2006 pp 813-838.

Bronchodilator drugs

Pesce AJ, Rashkin M, Kotagal U. Standards of laboratory practice: theophylline and caffeine monitoring. National Academy of Clinical Biochemistry. Clin Chem 1998; **44:** 1124-1128

Cardioactive drugs

Amiodarone

Campbell TJ, Williams KM. Therapeutic drug monitoring: antiarrhythmic drugs. Br J Clin Pharmacol 2001; **52 Suppl 1:** 21S-34S.

Freedman MD, Somberg JC. Pharmacology and pharmacokinetics of amiodarone. J Clin Pharmacol 1991; **31:** 1061-9.

Ursella S, Testa A, Mazzone M, Gentiloni SN. Amiodarone-induced thyroid dysfunction in clinical practice. Eur Rev Med Pharmacol Sci 2006; **10:** 269-78.

Digoxin

Gheorghiade M, van Veldhuisen DJ, Colucci WS. Contemporary use of digoxin in the management of cardiovascular disorders. Circulation 2006; **113:** 2556-64.

Morris RG, Jones TE, Goldsworthy SJ, Wagner TJ, Ho H, Horowitz JD. Suspected DLIS interference in the dimension DGNA digoxin assay method and the clinical application of the revised digoxin target range. Ther Drug Monit 2006; **28:** 454-7.

Rathore SS, Curtis JP, Wang Y, Bristow MR, Krumholz HM. Association of serum digoxin concentration and outcomes in patients with heart failure. JAMA 2003; **289:** 871-8.

Wu SL, Li W, Wells A, Dasgupta A. Digoxin-like and digitoxin-like immunoreactive substances in elderly people. Impact on therapeutic drug monitoring of digoxin and digitoxin concentrations. Am J Clin Pathol 2001; **115:** 600-4.

Drugs of abuse

Crettol S, Deglon JJ, Besson J. Croquette-Krokkar M, Gothuey I, Hammig R, *et al.* Methadone enantiomer plasma levels, CYP2B6, CYP2C19 and CYP2C9 genotypes and response to treatment. Clin Pharmacol Ther 2005; **78:** 593-604.

Elkader A, Sproule B. Buprenorphine: clinical; pharmacokinetics in the treatment of opioid dependence. Clin Pharmacokinet 2005; **44:** 661-680.

Gerger JG, Rhodes RJ, Gal J. Stereoselective metabolism of methadone N-demethylation by cytochrome P450 2B6 and 2C19. Chirality 2004; **16:** 36-44.

Immunosuppressive drugs

Ciclosporin

Johnston A, Chusney G, Schutz E, Oellerich M, Lee TD, Holt DW. Monitoring cyclosporin in blood: between-assay differences at trough and 2 hours post-dose (C2). Ther Drug Monit 2003; **25**: 167-73.

Johnston A, Belitsky P, Frei U, et al. Potential clinical implications of substitution of generic cyclosporine formulations for cyclosporine microemulsion (Neoral) in transplant recipients. Eur J Clin Pharmacol 2004; **60**: 389-95.

Levy G, Burra P, Cavallari A, *et al.* Improved clinical outcomes for liver transplant recipients using cyclosporine monitoring based on 2-hr post-dose levels (C2). Transplantation 2002; **73**: 953-9.

Morris RG, Holt DW, Armstrong VW, Griesmacher A, Napoli KL, Shaw LM. Analytic aspects of cyclosporine monitoring, on behalf of the IFCC/IATDMCT Joint Working Group. Ther Drug Monit 2004; **26**: 227-30.

Oellerich M, Armstrong VW, Kahan B, *et al.* Lake Louise Consensus Conference on cyclosporin monitoring in organ transplantation: report of the consensus panel. Ther Drug Monit 1995; **17**: 642-54.

Mycophenolate

Hesselink DA, van Gelder T. Genetic and nongenetic determinants of between-patient variability in the pharmacokinetics of mycophenolic acid. Clin Pharmacol Ther 2005; **78**: 317-21.

van Gelder T, Meur YL, Shaw LM, Oellerich M, DeNofrio D, Holt C, *et al.* Therapeutic drug monitoring of mycophenolate mofetil in transplantation. Ther Drug Monit 2006; **28**: 145-54.

van Hest RM, Hesselink DA, Vulto AG, Mathot RA, van Gelder T. Individualization of mycophenolate mofetil dose in renal transplant recipients. Expert Opin Pharmacother. 2006; **7**: 361-76.

van Hest RM, Mathot RA, Vulto AG, Ijzermans JN, van Gelder T. Within-patient variability of mycophenolic acid exposure: therapeutic drug monitoring from a clinical point of view. Ther Drug Monit 2006; **28**: 31-4.

Sirolimus

Buhaescu I, Izzedine H, Covic A. Sirolimus – Challenging current perspectives. Ther Drug Monit 2006; **28:** 577-584.

Holt DW, Denny K, Lee TD, Johnston A. Therapeutic monitoring of sirolimus: its contribution to optimal prescription. Transplant Proc 2003; **35 (3 Suppl):** 157S-161S.

Everolimus

Kovarik JM, Beyer D, Schmouder RL. Everolimus drug interactions: application of a classification system for clinical decision making. Biopharm Drug Dispos 2006; **27:** 421-426

Tacrolimus

Christians U, Jacobsen W, Benet LZ, Lampen A. Mechanisms of clinically relevant drug interactions associated with tacrolimus. Clin Pharmacokinet 2002; **41:** 813-851.

Ciancio G, Burke GW, Gaynor JJ, Ruiz P, Roth D, Kupin W, *et al.* A randomized long-term trial of tacrolimus/sirolimus versus tacrolimus/mycophenolate versus cyclosporine/sirolimus in renal transplantation: three-year analysis. Transplantation 2006; **81:** 845-852.

First MR. Tacrolimus based immunosuppression. J Nephrol 2004; **17 Suppl 8:** S25-31.

Chapter 3

Analytical aspects

Introduction

Establishment of a relationship between drug concentrations and effect requires accurate, precise and reliable methodologies. This requires no interference from endogenous compounds or from exogenous sources and it may also be necessary to detect pharmacologically active metabolites. Thus appropriate and robust analytical methods are the cornerstone of an effective TDM service.

Historically, early assays were colorimetric or based on measurement of UV absorbance e.g. monitoring salicylate therapy in patients with rheumatoid arthritis in the 1950s and 1960s using the Trinder method, or permanganate reduction of phenytoin and UV measurement of the solvent-extracted product. These methods lacked sensitivity and specificity, and were often cumbersome. Much of the pioneering work on the archetypal TDM drugs, the anticonvulsants, was done using gas or liquid chromatography. However, TDM was popularised with the ready availability of the EMIT methods in the early 1970s.

Since that time TDM analysis has undergone a revolution. The older, well-established drugs are assayed using a variety of immunoassays on general chemistry or immunoassay platforms, while more specialist assays have been developed for newer niche TDM drugs such as immunosuppressants, which utilise chromatography-mass spectrometry.

The principles of the main methods are considered below, and references at the end of this chapter give further details.

Selecting the most appropriate analytical methods is often not easy and the choice depends on the availability of staff, expertise and equipment, the nature of the service to be provided and the range of drugs to be assayed. The widely varying chemical nature of the substances measured for TDM purposes means that it is not possible to offer a comprehensive service based on a single analytical principle. Compromises have to be made between using the best method for each individual analyte, the ability to process samples within an appropriate time, the existing laboratory equipment profile and the use of techniques that allow quantitation of a wide range of substances.

The basic requirements of any method are that it should be accurate, precise, sufficiently sensitive and that the sample size should be acceptably small (certainly less than 1 mL plasma and ideally 10-100 μL). In addition, the method should be specific for the substance in question and free from interference from structurally related compounds or endogenous plasma components.

Assays based on colorimetry, fluorescence or UV absorbance of the analyte are no longer acceptable as routine analytical methods for TDM, though 'one-off' assays may require recourse to such an approach. For the vast majority of drugs which need to be assayed for the purposes of therapeutic drug monitoring, the choice lies between chromatographic methods and immunoassays. The exception is lithium, where historically atomic absorption or flame emission spectrometry were utilised and ion-selective electrodes are now preferred. The arguments between immunoassay and chromatographic procedures have been well rehearsed in a number of publications, and will only be summarized briefly here. The advantages and disadvantages of each are shown in Figure 3.1. In many senses they are complementary techniques rather than alternatives and the choice of which to use in a particular situation will depend on the information required, cost and available expertise.

Chromatography versus immunoassays for drug analysis

	Chromatography	Immunoassay
Applicability	Wide	Limited
Specificity	Yes	Sometimes
Speed	Slow - Medium	Slow - Fast
Capital cost	High	Low - High
Consumables cost	Low	Medium - High
Skill required (hence labour cost)	Medium - High	Low - Medium
Suitability for stat/clinic analysis	Poor	Good

Figure 3.1 Comparison between chromatography and immunoassay for drug analysis

Chromatographic methods

Chromatographic methods comprise several modes: Thin-Layer Chromatography (TLC), Gas Chromatography (GC) and Liquid Chromatography (LC). The attraction of such systems is their flexibility, enabling a wide range of different molecules to be analysed in a selective and quantitative manner, and their adaptability to a wide range of compounds. Most organic molecules can be separated and quantitated by means of suitable chromatographic systems. Specific methods for new compounds can be devised relatively quickly in many cases, in contrast to immunoassays, where development times may be significant, especially if a new antiserum must be raised. A range of related compounds can be analysed in a single chromatographic run, which has significant advantages when a number of drugs are prescribed together (e.g. anticonvulsants), or when there is a need for separate measurement of a drug and its active metabolites (e.g. tricyclic antidepressants). High sensitivity is attainable with the use of specific detection systems such as electrochemical or nitrogen detectors or mass spectrometers. The combination of sensitivity, specificity and flexibility means that chromatographic procedures are unsurpassed for toxicological applications and the early phase of evaluation of concentration-effect profiles for new drugs that may require TDM.

However, chromatographic methods do have some significant disadvantages. In comparison to immunoassays they are slow, labour intensive techniques which frequently demand a high degree of technical expertise to maintain efficient operation. Sample throughput is generally lower than for immunoassays – although this can be improved to some extent by partial or complete automation; the linear nature of column chromatographic analysis cannot compete with the rapidity of automated immunoassay for larger batches. Chromatographic data capture is readily interfacable with Laboratory Information Systems overcoming the previous reliance on data processors. However, the nature of calibration and variability inherent in chromatography and in the system means that ever greater sophistication is required than for mass-processing immunoassay analysers. Even greater numbers of analysts are turning to LC-tandem-MS because of the superior accuracy of the results and their inter-laboratory comparability, which allied with satisfactory data-handling enables routine use of such equipment. The capital cost of the equipment may be considerable, and the skilled labour required to develop and operate such systems has important revenue consequences. However, to monitor difficult compounds e.g. immunosuppressants and to establish 'gold standard' methods, chromatography combined with mass spectrometry is invaluable. Indeed liquid chromatography-tandem mass spectrometry is a viable option for routine applications at higher workloads.

Chromatographic methods usually require larger sample volumes than immunoassays, which is particularly relevant for paediatric applications. In addition, sample preparation is frequently more laborious, since extraction or formation of a chemical derivative may be required before the chromatographic step. Analysis time is thus lengthened, and this factor, together with the time required for a chromatograph to stabilize initially, makes chromatographic techniques less suitable when time is of the essence, for example in out-patient clinics or when results are needed urgently or outside normal laboratory hours. These factors have limited the application of chromatographic methods for routine TDM, despite their undoubted advantages.

The choice is normally between gas-liquid chromatography (GC) and high performance liquid chromatography (HPLC). The previously dominant position of GC has been eroded and is probably now only relevant if combined with mass spectrometric detection. HPLC and HPLC-MS are now the methods of choice for most (but not all) TDM applications where suitable immunoassays are not available.

Sample Preparation

Chromatography is not readily amenable to direct introduction of plasma to the chromatographic system due to the high protein concentration in plasma. The mode of chromatography may be such that a hydrophilic analyte may need to be concentrated to enable satisfactory detection concentrations or to be compatible with the chromatographic system. There are variations on the theme, but there are two main choices for sample preparation: liquid-liquid extraction (LLE) and liquid-solid extraction (LSE)/solid-phase extraction (SPE).

LIQUID–LIQUID EXTRACTION

An ionised compound is water soluble and lipophobic. To isolate it from an aqueous, proteinaceous sample requires extraction into an immiscible organic solvent, which requires the analyte to be made more lipophilic. This is achieved by ion-suppression e.g. for a basic drug the aqueous phase is made basic, for an acidic drug, acidic. The pH change needs to be > 2 pH units from the pK_a for the analyte. By evaporating the solvent, or using a concentrating aqueous to organic ratio, the analyte may be concentrated to a degree, enabling appropriate sensitivity for analysis. Back-extraction by reversing the pH change enables further sample clean-up. This is a labour intensive process requiring the use of potentially toxic and/or flammable solvents and its use is falling out of favour for these reasons. Experienced analysts can readily devise extraction strategies for new compounds with sufficient selectivity and sensitivity to enable detection of the analytes of interest. Sadly, such technical skill is now a rare commodity in clinical laboratories.

LIQUID-SOLID EXTRACTION

The sample is applied to a solid bed of resin, silica or selective phase modified silica. Typically the analyte is retained on the basis of its physicochemical properties: van der Waals forces, hydrogen bonding, ionic interaction or a combination of these, with the sample matrix being unretained. Selectivity is improved with carefully chosen elution solvents, with organic strength sufficient to attract the analyte away from the column bed but leaving behind more strongly retained interfering substances. The eluting solvent needs to be compatible with the chromatographic system.

INTERNAL STANDARDS

An internal standard is used in most chromatographic procedures to compensate for loss of material during sample preparation and chromatography. The underlying assumption is that losses of the internal standard during processing will be similar to losses of the analyte being measured and the internal standard must therefore be selected to have similar physicochemical properties to the analyte, i.e. it extracts at the same pH with the same yield as the analyte and has similar chromatographic properties. Injudicious selection of internal standards can adversely affect analytical performance.

Thin-Layer Chromatography

Despite some impressive examples of performance, high-performance thin-layer chromatographic techniques (HPTLC) have not found application in TDM laboratories. HPTLC has the distinct advantages of enabling parallel sample analysis and the ability to detect not only the parent drug, but also the full range of metabolites or a number of congeners. However, a good knowledge of the chemical properties of the analytes is required not only to effect separation, but also to devise a reaction system.

Gas-Liquid Chromatography (GC)

GC was the first technique with the required specificity to be used for TDM and formed the basis of the first reliable methods to evaluate and apply information on concentration and pharmacodynamic relationships. The requirement for volatility inherent in GC restricts its range of applicability. Originally the liquid phase was coated on to a solid phase support and columns were packed, but these have been replaced by capillary columns with a thin film of liquid phase on the column wall. These open-tubular columns have greater chromatographic efficiency and hence high resolving power.

GC is a cheap, flexible and precise method for the quantitation of drug molecules. Much of the early complexity of GC techniques has been removed with computer -controlled instruments with automatic temperature programming, data handling and autosampling. GC with flame-ionisation detection is the closest thing to a universal mass-sensitive detector, but more specific detection systems are available for particular applications (the nitrogen detector, and the electron-capture detector for halide-containing species). The ability to detect substances with no UV absorption and non-specific functional groups makes GC essential for some analytes, e.g. organic alcohols and volatile solvents.

GC is highly flexible, and methylsilicone columns such as DB-5 are applicable to the quantitation of a wide range of compounds. The major limitation of the technique is the requirement for analytes to be in the gas phase, which makes GC very useful for volatile substances but means that non-volatile compounds must be converted to more volatile derivatives before they can be subjected to chromatography. This involves chemical modification of polar residues like hydroxyl groups to prevent hydrogen bonding and lower the boiling point. The requirement for high temperatures also means that thermolabile compounds like carbamazepine and its 10,11-epoxide metabolite are difficult to chromatograph by GC. Capillary columns have reduced the need for derivatisation and have markedly improved resolving power and sensitivity.

Gas chromatography-mass spectrometry (GC-MS)

GC-MS bench-top systems are now readily affordable, though TDM work would need to be combined with other analyses e.g. drugs of abuse in most laboratories to allow economic use of the system. A skilful analyst is essential for successful utilisation of GC-MS. The need to modify polar groups by derivatisation contributes to the complexities of the compound libraries. While several thousand compounds are identifiable through libraries, the power of GC-MS is best utilised in TDM by using single ion monitoring, a technique where an abundant unique ion is monitored providing sensitivity and specificity. In electron impact (EI) MS, separation of the molecule of interest enables a skilled operator to determine the fragmentation pattern; from this examination putatative metabolites can be identified by calculating their fragmentation patterns against the parent and from this determining hydroxylation, demethylation etc. However, sometimes this approach can be time consuming. A gentler ionisation technique – chemical ionisation (CI) – yields a better molecular ion, but requires a knowledgeable operator for successful results. While liquid chromatography has greater flexibility than GC, particularly when linked to MS, temperature programmed capillary GC-MS will cover a wide spectrum of compounds, provided they are volatile or can be made so.

Liquid Chromatography

Liquid chromatography (LC), or more correctly, high performance liquid chromatography (HPLC), is the major chromatographic method used for therapeutic drug monitoring. Like GC, it is a rapid and efficient separation technique, but typically does not require derivatisation of the analyte. In addition, it is extremely flexible, as the mobile phase composition can be readily manipulated allowing fine adjustments to the chromatographic conditions to improve the resolution of particular compounds. Sample preparation for HPLC assays is dependent on the mode of LC to be used. The hydrophilic nature of reverse-phase LC eluants is compatible with simpler sample preparations than for GC. However, as stated earlier, GC has the advantage of having a universal detection system in the flame ionisation detector, while LC detectors have varying degrees of sensitivity.

Normal-phase HPLC is analogous to thin-layer chromatography with a polar stationary phase (silica) and non-polar solvents. In TDM we generally wish to separate polar drugs and metabolites, and in a normal-phase system the drug and its metabolites will elute with the least polar compound first followed by those compounds with increasing polarity. There are a number of disadvantages to normal-phase LC: solvents typically absorb in the low UV, are toxic, flammable and ion-exchange or suppression can be unpredictable. While ion-exchange would seem an obvious mode, since most drugs are ionised, in practice sample preparation is no easier than for normal-phase and separation mechanisms can be difficult to predict.

A non-polar stationary phase and a polar mobile phase (reverse-phase HPLC) has been the mainstay of LC for TDM purposes. Typically the stationary phase is silica with a C18 hydrocarbon chain chemically bonded to the surface, residual silanol groups are 'capped' with C2 to minimise silanol (normal-phase type) interactions. Suitably polar solvents include acetonitrile, methanol and aqueous buffers, or some combination of these. The advantages of reverse-phase are: compatibility with minimally prepared biological fluids, ready manipulation of ion-suppression and ready establishment and manipulation of dynamic ion-exchange systems using ion-pairing.

The selectivity of the mobile phase is critical to the accuracy of HPLC techniques, and careful evaluation of methods is essential before they are applied for routine purposes. Studies to detect possible interferences must be carried out with a wide range of commonly used drugs as well as endogenous metabolites, and when small changes to the mobile phase are made to improve the resolution of an established method, it is necessary to ensure that previously resolvable compounds do not now co-elute. Unfortunately, some methods in clinical use today have not been checked for interference even by closely related compounds. e.g. lack of resolution of theophylline and the structurally related caffeine metabolite 1,7-dimethylxanthine (paraxanthine); significant interference is possible if the two compounds are not resolved. In a survey of methods used by participants in the

UK External Quality Assessment Scheme for theophylline, it was noted that the use of mobile phases with lower proton donor selectivity values, i.e. those based on ethanol, methanol or tetrahydrofuran, appeared to increase the likelihood of achieving a separation.

Once an adequate separation of the compounds of interest has been achieved on the chromatographic column, it is necessary to detect and quantitate them in the column eluent. This is usually done by monitoring the ultraviolet absorbance of the eluent at a specific wavelength. The choice of monitoring wavelength for a range of compounds is necessarily a compromise. For example, the absorption maximum of carbamazepine is at approximately 280 nm, and this would be the optimum wavelength if this drug alone were being measured. However, other anticonvulsant drugs show no absorption at 280 nm, and a much shorter wavelength must be used to get adequate peaks for phenytoin and phenobarbitone. Acetonitrile, if suitably purified, allows monitoring of the UV absorption of the column effluent down to 190 nm, whereas methanol absorbs UV light below 210 nm and precludes the use of very low wavelength detection. The sensitivity of methanol-based or aqueous solvent systems is thus limited. It should be stressed that the UV detector is not a mass-sensitive detector, and careful external standardisation is required. Multiple wavelength monitoring can be achieved using linear diode arrays composed of a succession of diodes each sensitive to slightly different wavelengths, but these tend not to be as sensitive as monochromatic detectors.

Other detection systems include fluorescence and electrochemical detectors. These are not widely used for the majority of drugs, but are essential for some drug classes (for example the aminoglycoside antibiotics require fluorescence detection and morphine requires electrochemical detection). Drugs that have no specific functional groups or spectral properties (e.g. valproic acid) may sometimes be converted to compounds suitable for monitoring by pre-column or post-column derivatisation and conversion to a species with a discrete UV absorption maximum.

HPLC systems are particularly suitable for compounds which (because of their thermolabile nature or for other reasons) are unsuitable for GC analysis. These include the benzodiazepines, carbamazepine and its 10,11-epoxide. By its nature chromatography enables the simultaneous determination of a number of compounds and their metabolites. Sometimes this is achievable with isocratic elution, but it usually requires gradient elution. For example the anticonvulsant drugs phenytoin, phenobarbitone, carbamazepine, its 10,11-epoxide and lamotrigine can all be quantitated in a single run.

With the introduction of the immunosuppressant ciclosporin, sophisticated LC methods were developed. Identification of the complex metabolites requires MS. There are different types of MS: ion-trap and quadrapole with hybrids and varying geometries, these instruments are becoming more affordable with LC-MS-MS (LC-tandem MS) becoming the standard for certain assays e.g. sirolimus. The flexibility of MS and the bias inherent in some immunoassays has meant the adoption of LC-MS-MS for a number of immunosuppressant assays which are not amenable to standard LC methods, for reasons of lack of chromophore, sensitivity or sample preparation. LC-tandem MS can be utilised with minimal sample preparation and this has expanded the appeal of the technique. Indeed, the costs have now fallen to such a degree that it is possible to consider using LC-tandem MS for routine purposes instead of immunoassays.

Immunoassays

Immunoassays, as conventional separation radioimmunoassays, have been applied to the determination of therapeutic drugs since Oliver et al described a radioimmunoassay for digitoxin in 1968. However, the advent of homogeneous non-isotopic immunoassay systems in the mid 1970s in the form of EMIT (enzyme-multiplied immunoassay technique) proved to be the foundation stone for the widespread adoption of immunoassays for drugs in clinical laboratories. This technique is still widely used today. Conventional isotopic immunoassays have served clinical biochemists well in the past, but safety and ease-of-use considerations saw radioisotope assays fall out of favour in the 1980s and they are now rarely used.

The advantages of homogeneous (not requiring a separation step) non-isotopic assays for routine drug measurement are obvious. They are generally technically simple, require little operator skill, and are amenable to automation, permitting much higher sample throughputs than are possible with isotopic or chromatographic systems.

A bewildering variety of approaches have been described, based on the principle that the signal from a labelled molecule is modulated in some way by its immediate enviroment – specifically, by whether or not it is bound to antibody. This allows the determination of antibody occupancy – the basis of any immunoassay – by detecting the extent of signal modification. A comprehensive discussion of the techniques that have been used and their underlying principles is beyond the scope of this chapter, and specialised texts should be consulted. However, the major techniques currently in use for therapeutic drug monitoring will be described briefly.

ENZYME-MULTIPLIED IMMUNOASSAY (EMIT)

EMIT, developed by the Syva Company, is based upon the finding that the activity of an enzyme (glucose 6-phosphate dehydrogenase) chemically coupled to a drug molecule is inhibited when the drug is bound to a specific antibody, either because the substrate is sterically prevented from reaching the active site or because the close proximity of the antibody molecule induces conformational changes in the enzyme which distort the active site and prevent catalysis. After incubation of sample, enzyme-labelled drug and antibody, the substrate for the enzyme system is added and the reaction monitored by the conversion of NAD to NADH at 340 nm. The extent of enzyme activity reflects the proportion of enzyme-labelled drug which is not bound to antibody, which in turn reflects the number of binding sites occupied by unlabelled (sample) drug and hence the drug concentration in the sample (Figure 3.2). Since each labelled molecule can produce many product molecules, this system has a very high sensitivity, at least in theory. In practice, the sensitivity is limited by a relatively low signal to noise ratio and a limited dynamic range.

Enzyme multiplied immunoassay (EMIT)

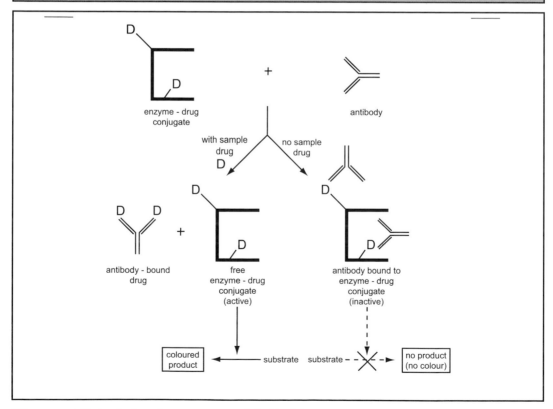

Figure 3.2 Principle of enzyme multiplied immunoassay (EMIT)

EMIT is easily applicable to a wide range of automated clinical analysers, requiring only a basic reagent addition system and a spectrophotometer with good temperature control and the ability to make multiple readings at 340nm. Kits are available for a wide range of drugs. Although the earliest of the homogenous assay systems it is still a widely used technique.

FLUORESCENCE POLARISATION IMMUNOASSAY (FPIA)

The technique of FPIA, originally described by Landon and coworkers and implemented commercially by Abbott Laboratories, is based on the relationship between the fluorescence lifetime of a labelled drug and its rotational relaxation time.

Drug labelled with a fluorophore (usually fluorescein) is excited by plane polarised light. If the drug conjugate is not bound to antibody, it can rotate freely in solution and rotation can occur between absorption of the incident light and fluorescence emission. This means that when the fluorescence photon is emitted, the molecule is no longer in the same orientation relative to the plane of polarisation, and the emitted fluorescence is not polarised in a single plane. By contrast, if the drug conjugate is bound to an antibody, the large size of the antibody molecule reduces its rotational relaxation time by approximately 100-fold. This means that little rotational movement of the antibody-drug conjugate is possible in the interval between absorption and emission of light, and the emitted light is polarised in the same plane as the incident light. The degree of depolarisation of the emitted fluorescence is therefore directly proportional to the amount of free conjugate. If labelled drug conjugate and sample drug are allowed to compete for a limited amount of antibody, the degree of depolarisation then reflects the sample drug concentration. The intensity of the polarised emission is inversely related to the sample drug concentration (Figure 3.3).

Since the technique requires polarisation filters and fluorescence optics, it is much less applicable to a range of analyzers. A very wide array of kits is available, covering the vast majority of drugs for which TDM is relevant.

Fluorescence polarisation immunoassay (FPIA)

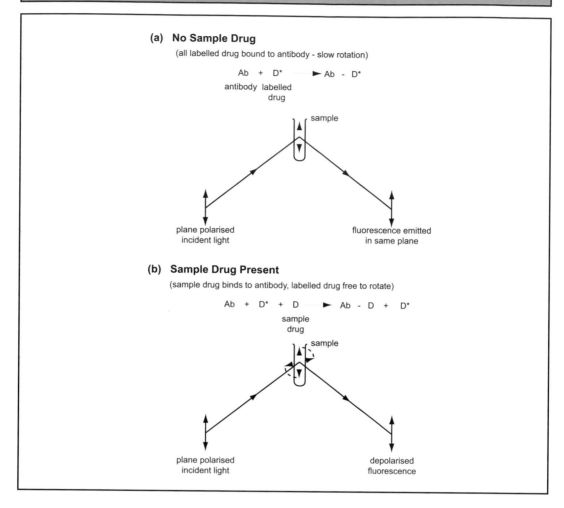

(a) No Sample Drug

(all labelled drug bound to antibody - slow rotation)

Ab + D* ► Ab - D*

antibody labelled
drug

sample

plane polarised
incident light

fluorescence emitted
in same plane

(b) Sample Drug Present

(sample drug binds to antibody, labelled drug free to rotate)

Ab + D* + D ► Ab - D + D*

sample
drug

sample

plane polarised
incident light

depolarised
fluorescence

Figure 3.3 Principle of fluorescence polarisation immunoassay (FPIA)

CEDIA

Cloned enzyme donor immunoassays (CEDIA) use recombinant DNA to produce inactive variants of the tetrameric enzyme beta-galactosidase in two complementary forms, an enzyme acceptor and an enzyme donor. These combine in solution to yield a functional enzyme. Binding of an antibody to the drug of interest to the enzyme donor inhibits this association. Thus the greater the amount of drug present the greater the free electron donor is available to combine with the electron acceptor (Figure 3.4). Clearly anything which disrupts this self-assembly will interfere in the assay. CEDIA assays are widely used on clinical chemistry analysers.

Cloned enzyme donor immunoassays (CEDIA)

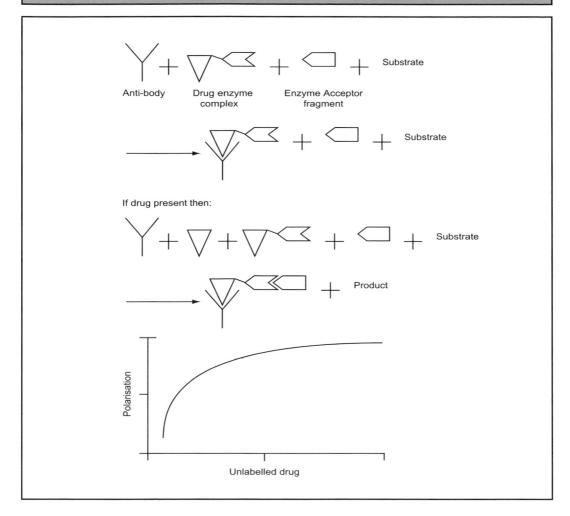

Figure 3.4 Principle of cloned enzyme donor immunoassay (CEDIA)

Chemiluminescence

If a chemiluminescent label is used to tag drug molecules, it is possible to construct assay geometries such that binding of antibody to antigen either enhances or inhibits the luminescent properties of the label, enabling discrimination between bound and free label. Stable dioxetanes are used as labels in the Immulite assays available from Siemens Medical Solutions Diagnostics.

Kinetic interaction of molecules in solution (KIMS)

In KIMS assays, the drug is bound to the surface of a microparticle; if there is no competing drug in a sample then the immobilised drug binds to the antibodies causing aggregates to form resulting in a change in light absorbance. If there is drug in the sample, it binds to the antibody and therefore less of the immobilised drug is bound and less light is transmitted; this is proportional to the concentration of the drug in the sample (Figure 3.5).

Kinetic interaction of molecules in solution (KIMS)

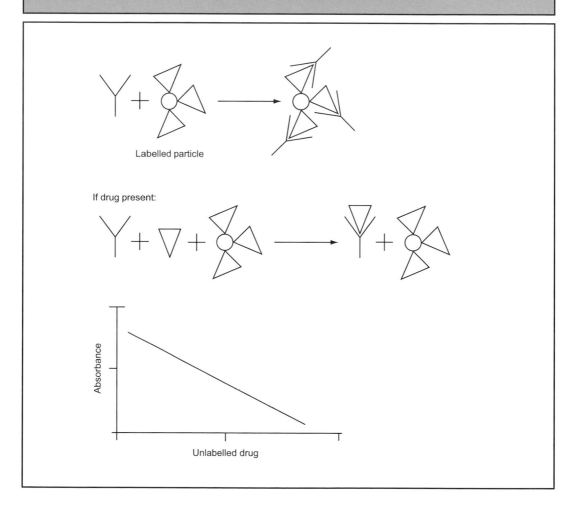

Figure 3.5 Principle of Kinetic Interaction of Molecules in Solution (KIMS) assays

Light scattering immunoassays

This term encompasses both turbidimetric and nephelometric assays. Essentially the combination of antigen and antibody forms an aggregate, which is large enough to scatter light. Turbidimetry is the measurment of the decrease in intensity of an incident beam of light that has passed through a solution. Forward angle nephelometry gives greater sensitivity, and is better for large molecule aggregates in dilute solution. Particle enhancement with e.g. latex particles has the benefit of improving sensitivity with greater light scattering, allowing the measurement of haptens such as drugs and decreasing the risk of antigen excess. These assays can be monitored as end-point or kinetic assays.

Dry Chemistry Systems and Thin-Film Immunoassays

So-called 'dry' reagent systems have considerable advantages for determination of drugs, such as convenience of reagent packaging, long shelf life, ease of disposal of potentially biohazardous waste and relative freedom from analytical interferences. However, although these approaches were popular in the 1980s and 1990s, their appeal has waned as TDM analysis has been incorporated into routine high-throughput clinical chemistry analysers. The Ortho-Clinical Diagnostics system is the only such system currently available using thin-film technology.

Enzyme inhibition assay

This system is not based on immunoassay, but will be mentioned here for completeness. Theophylline acts as a specific non-competitive inhibitor of beef liver alkaline phosphatase. A dry slide containing alkaline phosphatase and a chromogenic substrate is activated when sample is added, and the enzyme activity measured is inversely proportional to the theophylline present in the sample. This technique is obviously not applicable to a range of drugs, since it depends on a specific chemical property of theophylline.

Specificity of immunoassays

One of the major problems confronting the user of any immunoassay system is to discover what the system is actually measuring. The antibody used in the assay is potentially as specific as the receptor to which the drug binds *in vivo*, but (unless the analyst is extremely fortunate) the molecular structure of the active site of the antibody will not be the same as the molecular structure of the receptor, and their reactivity to compounds other than the one of interest may well differ significantly. This means that metabolites of drugs which are structurally similar to the parent drug may bind to the antibody and be measured in the immunoassay even though they do not bind to the receptor and are therefore biologically inactive. The reverse situation may also arise, e.g. for carbamazepine where the 10,11-epoxide is biologically active but not measured by most immunoassays. This factor may have a marked effect in reducing the observed correlation between apparent plasma drug concentration and clinical effect. Even when a metabolite is biologically active and recognised by the antibody, it is likely that the ratio of metabolite bioactivity to that of the parent compound will not be the same as the immunoactivity ratio, which adds further complexity to the situation. Drugs with a large number of metabolites with similar structures are a particular problem in this respect (e.g. benzodiazepines, ciclosporin). Similarly, structurally related drugs may cross-react in an immunoassay, typically less, often much less, than the target compound, but occasionally more. The recent development of the Dade Behring carbamazepine/10,11-epoxide assay, which measures both compounds, is a unique example of an immunoassay designed to reflect pharmacologically active drug and metabolite.

A particular example of the general problem which has attracted considerable attention in the past is the case of Digoxin-like Immunoreactive Substances (DLIS). DLIS were first demonstrated in the serum of a patient with renal impairment that contained a substance that cross-reacted with anti-digoxin antibodies. It soon became clear that this substance (or substances) was also present in other conditions including hypertension, liver disease, renal disease and pregnancy, and in premature neonates. The presence of this substance gives rise to measurable digoxin concentrations in patients not receiving the drug, and falsely high concentration measurements for patients on digoxin, which may result in misdiagnosis of digoxin toxicity. The presence of DLIS in patients with renal or hepatic failure is particularly problematical, as these are precisely the patients in whom digoxin monitoring is required.

The degree of interference observed with different immunoassays varies according to the specificity of the antibody in use. More recent assays have minimised DLIS interference, but the analyst must be aware of the potential problem and know the specificity and limitations of the particular method in use in his or her laboratory. Clinicians are usually unaware of such issues, and the experienced analyst has a vital role here.

Immunoassays – summary
The low technical skill requirements of immunoassays, their ready adaptability to automated systems and the availability of rapid results make them strong candidates for use in routine therapeutic drug monitoring. Against this must be set the specificity considerations outlined above, the relatively high reagent costs in comparison to chromatographic systems, especially when a range of analytes is to be determined on a single sample, and the fact that immunoassays are generally more susceptible to non-specific interference from endogenous components (haemoglobin, bilirubin, etc.) in the sample. These interferences can affect the antibody-antigen reaction itself or the efficiency of the detection system.

Immunoassays have higher development costs than chromatographic systems, and the development of sophisticated homogeneous non-isotopic systems is now virtually exclusively carried out by large commercial organisations. This is reflected in the higher revenue costs.

Chromatography or immunoassay?

Consolidation of TDM assays onto chemistry analysers often reduces overall cost (despite the higher cost per test), enhances ease of assay and enables a 'single-pass' analysis. Immunoassays have undoubted weaknesses, as detailed above, but speed of analysis and increased throughput does make them attractive options for the routine laboratory. Chromatography on the other hand is more demanding of user time and skills. It is therefore confined to developing areas of TDM or for esoteric assays. However, the simplicity and sensitivity of LC-MS-MS may challenge this view in the future. Providers of high volume immuno-suppressant monitoring services using immunoassay are switching to LC-MS-MS. The high initial capital costs can be recouped over a few years with low revenue costs. Such an approach will undoubtedly improve the accuracy of TDM analyses.

Chirality

Many pharmacologically active compounds contain a carbon atom linked to four different substituents, and thus have the potential to exist in two differently handed forms. This property is called chirality (from the Greek for hand) and the pair of mirror-image compounds are called stereoisomers (or enantiomers). Frequently, only one stereoisomer possesses the desired pharmacological action, and the other may be inactive or be active in a different way. For example, the D-isomer of propoxyphene is a narcotic analgesic whereas the L-isomer has no narcotic properties and is used as a cough suppressant. Stereoisomers may also show marked differences in pharmacokinetic parameters such as clearance and volume of distribution, and stereospecific analytical methods are required if meaningful conclusions are to be drawn in such cases. For example, the overall clearance of vigabatrin in children increases with age, suggesting that age-related dosing is necessary. However, stereoselective studies show clearly that clearance increases with age for only one isomer, and that isomer is inactive. The clearance of the active form is independent of age, and age-related dosing is unnecessary. The analytical approaches for stereospecific drug monitoring rely on HPLC. Immunoassays are of little use, because while the antibody used in the assay may well respond differently to the different isomeric forms, this is unlikely to reflect the different response of the receptor *in vivo*, which therefore adds further complexity to the situation.

No chiral drugs are routinely monitored by TDM services, though monitoring of D-amphetamine prescribed to amphetamine users discriminates illicit use of racemic street amphetamine. The expectation that the application of stereospecific methods would produce an entirely new crop of valid concentration-effect relationships for single enantiomers of chiral drugs and extend the clinical role for TDM has not been fulfilled. What has happened instead is that the pharmaceutical companies have increasingly selected enantiomers for their specific properties; one of the tragedies of thalidomide is that one enantiomer is reported to have caused the disastrous teratogenic effects which led to the drug being withdrawn, while the other had valuable pharmacological properties.

Free drug monitoring

The reasons for wishing to measure the amount of free (non-protein-bound) drug in biological fluids were outlined in Chapter 1, and only the analytical considerations will be discussed briefly here.

The three main methods for separation of bound and free drug prior to quantitation by conventional assays are equilibrium dialysis, ultrafiltration and centrifugation. Equilibrium dialysis involves the use of a dialysis chamber containing a semi-permeable membrane which allows the passage of low molecular weight species. Diluted plasma is placed within the membrane, and drug-free buffer outside it. Free drug then equilibrates between the two compartments, while bound drug is confined to the inner compartment. Quantitation of the drug concentration in the buffer compartment provides a measure of the free drug concentration in the sample.

Ultrafiltration and centrifugation are non-equilibrium techniques and are therefore much faster than equilibrium dialysis, which generally requires an overnight incubation. Both involve passing the sample through a fine-mesh filter or membrane. Micro-separation devices are commercially available. A disadvantage with ultrafiltration and centrifugation techniques in comparison with equilibrium dialysis is that it is more difficult to control the temperature and pH of the separation, which may have significant effects on the degree of protein binding and thus the observed free concentration of the drug. On the other hand, the dilution of drug which inevitably occurs during equilibrium dialysis, may alter concentration-dependent binding equilibria. Another potential problem affecting all the techniques is loss of drug by adsorption on to the membrane or filter used for separation. It is often difficult to assess the reliability of different procedures as no single method consistently gives accurate estimates of free drug concentrations. Thus, many investigators compare the results of two or more techniques when evaluating new methods or new drugs.

For drugs predominantly bound to albumin (e.g. phenytoin), calculated 'free' drug concentrations can be obtained that are a reasonable approximation e.g. phenytoin. However, basic drugs are bound to other proteins such as α_1-acid glycoprotein, which is rarely (if ever) measured and no calculated 'free' drug formulae are used in practice.

Attempts to introduce free drug monitoring into routine practice in the UK have generally been unsuccessful, yet it is not uncommon in the best US centres. The reasons for this are partly related to cost and partly to lack of understanding by both laboratory staff and clinicians.

Salivary monitoring
An alternative approach to determining free drug concentrations is to use an *in vivo* ultrafiltrate i.e. to use saliva as the sample. The majority of drugs enter saliva from plasma by passive diffusion of unbound non-ionised drug down a concentration gradient at a rate proportional to saliva flow rate and dependent upon their degree of ionisation. Drug concentrations in saliva reflect plasma free drug concentrations quite well for drugs which are largely unionised at physiological pH, e.g. phenytoin. Salivary monitoring is unsuitable for drugs that are actively secreted into saliva (e.g. lithium) and drugs that are strongly ionised at physiological pH (e.g. valproic acid, quinidine).

If saliva is to be used, it is important to establish the extent of binding of the drugs to be studied to mucoprotein and cellular debris present in the sample, because centrifugation of the sample will separate this material from the free drug in the supernatant. For several anticonvulsant drugs (e.g. phenobarbitone and carbamazepine) it has been demonstrated that no binding to salivary proteins occurs.

Careful collection of the sample is invariably required, and this involves thorough cleansing of the mouth with water before sampling. Sapid or masticatory stimulation of saliva flow is used to increase saliva volume and causes a significant increase in pH from around 6.8 to 8, which will affect the saliva/plasma partition ratio. Collection and analysis of saliva samples poses aesthetic problems for both patients and laboratory staff, which accounts to some extent for the limited use of the technique. The mucoproteins in saliva make samples difficult to handle and pipette accurately, and centrifugation is time-consuming and not completely effective in removing debris. Salivary analysis has some merit for phenytoin and carbamazepine estimations in small children where blood sampling may be difficult, but has not been widely adopted.

Quality assurance

It is self-evident that measurements of plasma drug concentrations can only be effectively used to diagnose toxicity or underdosage and to monitor treatment if such measurements are accurate and reproducible. The need for effective internal quality control and external quality assessment procedures is therefore as great as in other areas of clinical biochemistry. In TDM, where one may wish to estimate half-lives or times to steady state, analytical imprecision has a multiplicative effect on pharmacokinetic estimates.

The procedures used for quality assessment of drug assays are in general no different from those used for other analytes, and have been reviewed by Williams. A UK External Quality Assurance Scheme (UKNEQAS) is operated from the University Hospital of Wales, Cardiff (the Heathcontrol scheme provided by Cardiff Bioanalytical Services). Aminoglycoside antibiotics are covered by a scheme provided from Southmead Hospital, Bristol, UK and an internationally recognised scheme for immunosuppressants is offered from St George's Hospital, London, now under the UKNEQAS umbrella. TDM schemes are in operation in many other countries and are also provided by commercial agencies such as Randox and BioRad. Data collected from the Heathcontrol scheme have been used to assess the performance of various analytical techniques.

Units

While clinical chemistry laboratories changed over to molar SI units in the 1970s this did not uniformly occur for drugs, the specialist toxicology laboratories being particularly resistant. Debate ebbed and flowed with a roughly 50:50 split scattered around the UK. The reason for the desire to remain in mass units was grounded in the fact that in toxicology the molecular weight of rarely analysed drugs was not readily to hand and also much of the available data was from the USA, which still universally retained mass units.

In the UK the first move to uniformity was the publication of the joint National Poisons Information Service/Association of Clinical Biochemistry Guidelines on Laboratory Analyses for the poisoned patient [Ann Clin Biochem, **39:** 328-339; 2002]. With increasing networking of laboratory services and the establishment of shared electronic patient records it was becoming clear some consensus was needed. A consensus meeting of: Association for Clinical Biochemistry, Royal College of Physicians, Royal College of Pathologists, National Poisons Information Service, Association of Clinical Pathologists, Forensic Science Service and the International Association of Therapeutic Drug Monitoring and Clinical Toxicology agreed the use of mass SI units i.e. per litre for nearly all compounds except a specified few that have universally been reported in molar units: methotrexate, lithium, thyroxine, iron and units enshrined in legislation [Watson

& Barth ACB News **522:** 14-15; 2006]. The debate highlighted demonstrable risks to patients as identified by NPIS, making the case for uniformity vital.

A UK consensus in favour of SI mass units with the litre as the unit of volume has now been achieved.

Further reading

Armstrong VW, Shipkova M, von Ahsen N, Oesllerich M. Analytic aspects of monitoring therapy with thiopurine medications. Ther Drug Monit **26:** 220-226; 2004.

Ducharme J, Fernandez C, Gimenez F, Farinotti R. Critical issues in chiral drug analysis in biological fluids by high-performance liquid chromatography. J Chrom B: Biomedical Applications **668:** 65-75; 1996

Flanagan RJ, Taylor AA, Watson ID, Whelpton R. Fundamentals of Analytical Toxicology. John Wiley & sons 2008.

Gorodischer R, Koren G. Salivary excretion of drugs in children: theoretical and practical issues in therapeutic drug monitoring. Develop Pharmacol & Ther **19:** 161-177; 1992.

Martinavarro-Dominguez A, Capella-Peiro ME, Gil-Agusti M, Marcos-Tomas JV, Esteve-Romero J. Therapeutic drug monitoring of anticonvulsant drugs by micellar HPLC with difrect injection of serum samples. Clin Chem **48:** 1696-1702; 2002.

Pederen-Bjergaard S, Rasmussen KE. Bioanalysis of drugs by liquid-phase microextraction coupled to separation techniques. J Chrom B: Analytical Technologies in the Biomedical & Life Sciences. **817:** 3-12, 2005.

Steimer W, Muller C, Eber B. Digoxin assays: frequent, substantial and potentially dangerous interference with spironolactone, canrenone and other steroids. Clin Chem **48:** 507-516; 2002.

Steimer W, Zopf K, von Amelunxen S, Pfeiffer H, Bachofer J, Popp J *et al*, Amitriptyline or not, that is the question: pharmagenetic testing of CYP2D6 and CYP2C19 identifies patients with low or high risk for side effects in amitriptyline therapy. Clin Chem **51:** 376-385; 2005.

Sternson LA. The application of chemical derivatization to clinical drug analysis. Xenobiotica **17**: 385-396; 1987.

Thormann W. Progress of capillary electrophoresis in therapeutic drug monitoring and clinical and forensic toxicology. Ther Drug Monit **24**: 222-231; 2002.

Trtic-Petrovic T, Jonsson JA. Determination of drug-protein binding using supported liquid membrane extraction under equilibrium conditions. J Chrom B: Analytical Technologies in the Biomedical & Life Sciences. **814**: 375-384; 2005.

Tsai TH. Assaying protein unbound drugs using microdialysis techniques. J Chrom B: Analytical Technologies in the Biomedical & Life Sciences. **797**: 161-173, 2003.

Watson ID, HPLC for therapeutic drug monitoring and determination of toxicity. Adv Chromatog **26**: 117-189; 1987.

Wilson JF, Watson ID, Williams J, Toseland PA, Thomson AH, Sweeney G *et al*. Primary standardization of assays for anticonvulsant drugs: comparison of accuracy and precision. Clin Chem **48**: 1963-1969; 2002.

Witte DL. Matrix effects in therapeutic drug monitoring surveys. Proposed protocol to identify error components and quality improvement opportunities. Arch Pathol Lab Med **117**: 373-380; 1993

Chapter 4

Dosage prediction – Principles and practice

The initial chapters of this book have shown that therapeutic drug monitoring can play an important part in optimising drug therapy, especially in cases where clinical assessment of drug efficacy or toxicity is impossible. The dosage regime to achieve a desired concentration (which may not necessarily be within the target range) and hence a desired therapeutic effect can be predicted using the pharmacokinetic principles outlined in Chapter 1, provided that adequate clinical, biochemical and pharmacological data are available. This chapter discusses some of the approaches to dosage prediction that are available, and illustrates these with various case studies.

Pharmacokinetic principles

A number of key terms and equations form the basis of pharmacokinetics and dosage prediction. These were defined in Chapter 1 and include:

Bioavailability (page 5)

Unless a drug is given intravenously, not all of it reaches the bloodstream. The bioavailability (F) is the fraction of administered dose which reaches the systemic circulation.

Salt conversion factor (page 7)

Drugs may be administered as derivatives of their active form (e.g. salts or chelates). The salt conversion factor (S) is the fraction of active drug present in the compound administered. It follows that (from page 7):

$$\text{Amount of active drug reaching circulation} = S \times \text{Dose} \times F \qquad \text{Eq. 4.1}$$

A patient is given a single 300 mg tablet of quinidine sulphate. How much quinidine will appear in the circulation?

Salt conversion factor for quinidine sulphate (S) = 0.82
Bioavailability for quinidine (F) = 0.73

Dose reaching circulation = S x F x Dose
= 0.82 x 0.73 x 300
= 180 mg

Example 1

Rate of administration

The average rate at which a drug reaches the systemic circulation is termed the Rate of Administration (RA) and is calculated by dividing the amount of active drug reaching the bloodstream (see Eq. 1) by the time over which the drug was administered. For oral dosing, the time over which the drug was administered is conventionally taken to be the time between doses – the dosage interval, τ, even though absorption of the dose may be completed well before the next dose.

$$\text{Rate of Administration} = \frac{\text{Drug reaching circulation}}{\text{Time between doses}}$$

$$= \frac{S \times F \times \text{Dose}}{\tau} \qquad \text{Eq. 4.2}$$

A patient is given 300 mg aminophylline intravenously every 12 h. What is the average rate of administration of theophylline?

Salt conversion factor for aminophylline (S) = 0.8
Bioavailability for aminophylline (F) = 1.0
Dosage interval τ = 12 h

$$\text{Rate of administration} = \frac{0.8 \times 1.0 \times 300}{12}$$

$$= 20 \text{ mg/h}$$

Example 2

Volume of distribution (page 7)

The apparent volume of distribution (V_d) is defined as the volume of fluid necessary to contain the total amount of drug in the body if it were present throughout at a concentration equal to the plasma drug concentration. It can vary more than a thousand fold between different drugs, depending on the drug's water and lipid solubilities and the degree of plasma protein or tissue binding.

The amount of drug present in the body at a given time (t) after dosing is thus (by definition) $V_d \times C_p$, where C_p is the plasma concentration at time t. If plasma concentrations measured at various times after dosing can be back-extrapolated to the theoretical plasma concentration at the time of administration assuming instantaneous absorption and distribution (C_0), the volume of distribution may be estimated from:

$$\text{Volume of distribution} = \frac{\text{Dose absorbed}}{\text{Plasma concentration at time 0}}$$

$$= \frac{\text{S x F x Dose}}{C_0} \qquad \text{Eq. 4.3}$$

More precise methods for determining V_d involve multiple blood samples across the dosage interval and calculations based on the area under the concentration/time curve (AUC).

Loading Dose

The loading dose is the dose of drug given at the start of therapy to achieve an effective plasma concentration as rapidly as possible. If the volume of distribution of the drug in a given patient is known (or can be estimated from population data), the loading dose required to achieve a given plasma concentration may be estimated from a re-arranged equation 4.3:

$$\text{Dose} = \frac{C_0 \times V_d}{S \times F} \qquad \text{Eq. 4.4}$$

If there is drug already present in the circulation and it is desired to increase the concentration by a certain amount, Eq. 4.4 may also be used by substituting the desired concentration increment for C_0. It is important to remember that such calculations always assume instantaneous absorption and distribution of drug, which is obviously not the case in practice. If absorption is relatively rapid and distribution is slow (as is the case for digoxin, for example), administration of the calculated loading dose all at once may result in dangerously high concentrations of the drug in the plasma before it has a chance to distribute through the body. For this reason, loading doses may be divided into two or more separate amounts, administered some time apart.

Clearance (page 9)

Clearance (Cl) is the pharmacokinetic parameter which describes elimination of drug from the body, via the kidneys, liver, gut, lungs or skin. The clearance of a drug is defined as the theoretical volume of blood that could be completely cleared of drug in unit time. The rate of elimination of a drug is therefore given by multiplying the volume of blood that can be cleared of a drug in unit time (clearance) by the concentration of the drug:

$$\text{Rate of elimination} = \text{Clearance x Plasma concentration}$$

$$= Cl \times C_p \qquad \text{Eq. 4.5}$$

An 80 kg man has a trough plasma digoxin concentration of 0.5 µg/L (0.64 nmol/L). Assuming a normal volume of distribution, what oral loading dose would be required to obtain a plasma concentration of 1.5 µg/L (1.9 nmol/L)?

Salt conversion factor for digoxin = 1.0
Bioavailability for digoxin tablets = 0.62
Volume of distribution for digoxin = 7.3 L/kg = 7.3 x 80 = 584 L

From equation 4.4:

$$\text{Loading dose} = \frac{(C_{desired} - C_{initial}) \times V_d}{S \times F}$$

$$= \frac{(1.5 - 0.5) \times 584}{1.0 \times 0.62}$$

$$= 942 \; \mu g$$

In practice, 1 mg would be given, probably divided as two doses of 0.5 mg.

Example 3

At steady state on an established dose regime, the rate of administration of a drug equals the rate of elimination, and therefore (combining equations 4.2 and 4.5):

$$\text{Rate of administration} = \text{Rate of elimination}$$

$$\frac{S \times F \times Dose}{\tau} = Cl \times C_p$$

$$Cl = \frac{S \times F \times (Dose/\tau)}{C_p} \qquad \text{Eq. 4.6}$$

Clearance can be affected by a number of factors, including body size (see Figure 1.4). Values for clearance are often quoted as mL/min/kg body weight, but more accurate comparisons between patients are provided by expressing clearances in terms of body surface area. Surface areas can be determined from standard nomograms (see Appendix, Figures 1 & 2) or estimated from body weight using the formula:

$$\text{Body surface area (m}^2) = (\text{Weight in kg}/70)^{0.73} \times 1.73 \qquad \text{Eq. 4.7}$$

The two major routes of drug removal from the body are renal excretion and metabolism by the liver. They are generally assumed to be independent of one another and additive, so:

$$\text{Total clearance} = \text{Renal excretion} + \text{Hepatic metabolism}$$

Clearance measurements are more often adjusted for renal impairment than for hepatic impairment, in part because hepatic function is more difficult to measure. However, it is important to remember that both metabolic and renal clearance may be severely compromised when cardiac output declines. This is important in congestive cardiac failure, when hepatic clearance of digoxin and theophylline may fall by 50%. Liver enzymes may also be induced by alcohol or other drugs (e.g. anticonvulsants), and hepatic clearance will be increased in these circumstances.

Most clinical estimates of renal clearance are based on creatinine clearance, which may be calculated by concurrent assessment of plasma creatinine and creatinine excretion in an accurately timed urine specimen and calculation of creatinine clearance from the expression:

$$\text{Creatinine clearance} = \frac{U \times V}{P \times t} \qquad \text{Eq. 4.8}$$

where U and P represent urine and plasma concentrations, respectively (both in the same units) and V is the volume of urine produced over time t.

Clinical decisions may need to be taken rapidly, before a formal estimate of the creatinine clearance can be made. Because of this, and because accurate urine collections are often difficult to obtain, it may be more practical to estimate creatinine clearance or glomerular filtration rate (GFR) from the plasma creatinine concentration using the Cockcroft-Gault equation or Modified Diet in Renal Disease (MDRD) equations:

Cockcroft-Gault:

$$\text{Creatinine clearance (mL/min)} = \frac{S \times (140 - A) \times W}{P} \qquad \text{Eq. 4.9}$$

where S = 1.00 for women and 1.23 for men, A = age in years and W = ideal body weight in kg (unless this is greater than actual weight when actual weight should be used). This equation was derived from data on adults aged between 18 and 92 and should not be used for children or when renal function is unstable (i.e. creatinine production and excretion are not at steady state). A formula designed for children was reported by Schwartz *et al* and a nomogram for use in adults is also available (see Appendix Figure 3).

MDRD:

(abbreviated form, adapted for molar units):

$$GFR = 173 \times [S_{cr}]^{-1.154} \times [Age]^{-0.203} \times [0.742 \text{ if female}] \times [1.21 \text{ if patient is black}]$$

where S_{cr} represents serum creatinine in µmol/L and age is in years.

N.B. This form of the MDRD equation can only be used with creatinine methods that have been calibrated to be traceable to ID-MS reference methods. Variant forms of the equation are in use in the UK, related to different methods for creatinine determination. Readers should consult appropriate literature to determine that they are using the appropriate factor for a particular creatinine method.

Two compartment models

The simplest representation of the body as a vehicle for drug handling is to imagine it as a single pool in which all drugs are distributed and from which all drugs are cleared. This assumption has been implicit in the discussion above, and is known as the one compartment model. However, there are a number of situations in which this is inappropriate, and it is necessary to use a more physiologically realistic model in which the body is considered as having two (or, occasionally, more) compartments.

The first compartment, comprising the bloodstream and areas with a high blood flow, is termed the initial volume (V_i), and the second, representing areas where drug is slower to distribute, the tissue volume (V_t). Clearly,

$$V_d = V_i + V_t \qquad \text{Eq. 4.10}$$

For drugs which conform to this model, rapid administration of a loading dose into a small initial volume may result in higher early concentrations than predicted using the total volume of distribution. The consequences of this depend on whether target receptors, either for clinical effect or toxicity, behave as though they are located in the initial or tissue volumes.

If drugs exert their effects at sites in V_i , for example lignocaine and quinidine, toxicity may occur, and in such circumstances loading doses should be given slowly or in divided doses. When the target receptor is in V_t , as is the case for digoxin, plasma concentrations measured before distribution is complete will overestimate the active concentration and are therefore unreliable for predicting efficacy or toxicity.

For a two-compartment model, the concentration-time profile in V_i (the plasma concentration) after drug administration is shown in Figure 4.1. The figure illustrates the biphasic decay in two-compartment systems, the initial α half-life representing distribution into the tissues and the subsequent longer, β half-life representing elimination from V_i.

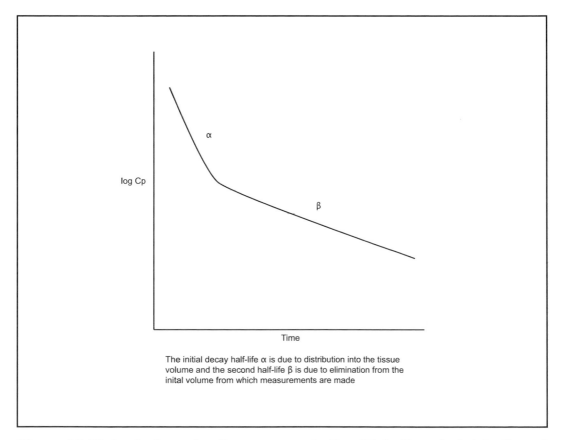

The initial decay half-life α is due to distribution into the tissue volume and the second half-life β is due to elimination from the inital volume from which measurements are made

Figure 4.1 Biphasic decay in plasma concentration (Cp) after administration of a drug exhibiting distribution kinetics consistent with a two compartment model.

A 70 year old woman was seen by her Family Doctor at a 9.30 am appointment. She had a one week history of feeling tired and nauseated and was on long-term digoxin, 0.125 mg daily. A blood sample taken for various biochemical tests including digoxin was received in the laboratory at 11.30 am.The digoxin result was 3.0 µg/L (3.9 nmol/L) – the target range for digoxin is 0.8 - 2.0 µg/L (1.0 - 2.6 nmol/L).

What comments should be made when the result is reported?

Most patients take their digoxin first thing in the morning, and it is likely that only 2 - 3 hours may have elapsed between dose and sampling. Because of digoxin's small initial volume of distribution and long α phase, blood samples should be taken at least six hours after dosing to ensure that the drug has had time to diffuse into the second compartment and reported plasma concentrations are not inappropriately high. If the dose was taken in the early morning the concentration of 3.0 µg/L cannot be interpreted and a further blood sample should be obtained at an appropriate time. It is also helpful to analyse the sample for potassium and creatinine concentrations – clinical digoxin toxicity may occur at concentrations within the target range when hypokalaemia is present, and renal function is a major determinant of digoxin clearance.

A sample taken the following day, 8 hours post-dose, gave a plasma digoxin concentration of 2.0 µg/L (2.6 nmol/L); plasma potassium concentration was 5.0 mmol/L and creatinine 125 µmol/L.

If patients took their digoxin in the late evening, such problems with sampling (which are very common) would be unlikely to occur.

Case study 1

Maintenance dose

Once therapy is established, either with or without a loading dose, the dose required to maintain any desired average plasma concentration (C_p) at steady state (the maintenance dose) may be derived from a rearrangement of equation 4.6:

$$\text{Maintenance dose} = \frac{C_p \times Cl \times \tau}{S \times F}$$

Eq. 4.11

If the drug clearance is known, either from population values in the literature or calculated for the individual patient, the maintenance dose can be calculated.

A man weighing 70 kg requires intravenous phenobarbital to be given by an 8 hourly regime. What dose is required to maintain an average steady state plasma concentration of 23.2 mg/L (100 μmol/L)? The mean value for clearance in a group of similar individuals was 4 mL/h/kg.

Required steady state concentration = 23.2 mg/L
Population clearance for phenobarbital = 4mL/h/kg. For a body weight of 70 kg this gives an estimated clearance of 0.28 L/h.
Dosage interval = 8 h
Salt conversion factor and bioavailability = 1.0

From equation 4.11,

$$\text{Maintenance dose} = \frac{23.2 \times 0.28 \times 8}{1.0}$$

$$= 52.0 \text{ mg} \quad \text{(i.e. 50 mg tds in practice)}$$

Example 4

First order kinetics

Drug elimination from the body frequently follows log-linear or first-order kinetics, in which a constant fraction of drug is removed whatever the concentration, and the plot of the logarithm of the plasma concentration against time is a straight line (Figure 4.2). The fraction of drug removed per unit time is termed the elimination rate constant (k_{el}) and the time taken for the drug concentration to fall to half of the initial concentration is the half-life, $t_{1/2}$.

First order drug elimination is described by:

$$C_t = C_0 \times e^{-k_{el}t} \qquad \text{Eq. 4.12}$$

Or

$$\ln C_t = \ln C_0 - k_{el}t \qquad \text{Eq. 4.13}$$

where C_0 and C_t are the plasma concentations at time zero and time t, respectively and the exponential term is the fraction of drug remaining at time t. In first order kinetics, both the volume of distribution and clearance are independent of the plasma concentration and changes in drug concentration are linearly related to fractional changes in dose.

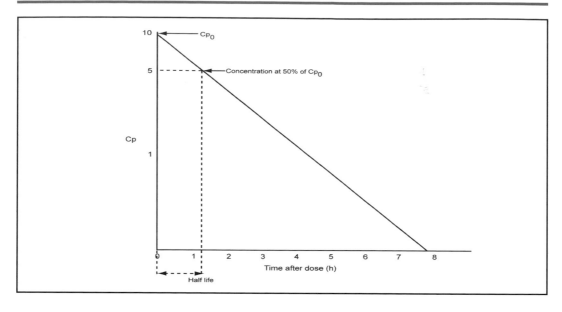

Figure 4.2 In first order elimination there is a logarithmic fall in plasma concentration or amount of drug within the body. Plotting concentration on a log scale versus time therefore gives a straight line and the half-life can easily be assessed as shown above

The patient in example 4 is given 25 mg phenobarbital rather than 52 mg every 8 hours. What is the new average steady state concentration (C_{ss})?

$$\text{New } C_{ss} \quad = \quad \text{Old } C_{ss} \quad \times \quad \text{Fractional change in dose}$$

$$= \quad 23.2 \quad \times \quad (25/52)$$

$$= \quad 11.2 \text{ mg/L}$$

This can be confirmed by rearranging equation 11:

$$C_{ss} \quad = \quad \frac{S \times F \times (\text{Dose}/\tau)}{Cl} \qquad \text{Eq. 14}$$

$$= \quad \frac{1.0 \times (25/8)}{0.28}$$

(clearance = 0.28 L/h, from example 4)

$$= \quad 11.2 \text{ mg/L}$$

Example 5

Elimination rate constant

It can be seen from Eq. 4.13 that the elimination rate constant k_{el} is the downward slope of the line obtained when the natural logarithm of plasma concentration is plotted against time. If common logarithms ($\log_{10}$) are used, as in Figure 4.2, then:

$$\log_{10} C_t \quad = \quad \log_{10} C_0 \quad \frac{k_{el}t}{2.303} \qquad \text{Eq. 4.15}$$

where 2.303 is ln 10, the proportionality constant between natural and common logarithms. A patient-specific value for the elimination rate constant can be obtained from two drug concentration measurements at known times during the elimination phase. For levels C_1 and C_2 taken at times t_1 and t_2 after dosing:

$$k_{el} \quad = \quad \ln (C_1/C_2)/(t_1 - t_2) \qquad \text{Eq. 4.16}$$

As shown in Chapter 1, page 11, the elimination rate constant can also be expressed in terms of clearance and volume of distribution.

$$k_{el} \quad = \quad \frac{\text{Amount of drug cleared in unit time}}{\text{Total amount in body}}$$

$$= \quad \frac{Cl \times C_p}{V_d \times C_p}$$

(see Eq. 5 and the definition of V_d above)

$$= \quad \frac{Cl}{V_d} \qquad \text{Eq. 4.17}$$

Half-life

In clinical situations, the elimination rate constant is usually expressed as the half-life ($t_{1/2}$). As shown in Figure 4.2, this is the time taken for the plasma concentration, or total body content, to fall by 50% and is related to k_{el} by the expression:

$$t_{1/2} \quad = \quad \frac{0.693}{k_{el}} \qquad \text{Eq. 4.18}$$

where 0.693 = ln 2. (see chapter 1 Eq. 1.10 for derivation of Eq. 4.18)

For drugs exhibiting first order kinetics, k_d and $t_{1/2}$ have a number of useful clinical applications such as predicting the time taken to reach steady state or to eliminate drug from the body, deciding the optimal dosage interval and calculating plasma concentrations for a variety of dosage regimes.

Time to steady state

After initiation or increase of a maintenance dose, drugs accumulate in the body until the amount eliminated equals that absorbed during each dosage interval. The patient is then said to be at steady state. The time taken to attain steady state is related to the elimination half-life of the drug – it takes one half-life to reach 50% of steady state concentration, two half-lives to reach 75%, three half-lives to reach 87.5%, four half-lives to reach 93.7% and five half-lives to reach 96.8%. For clinical purposes, effective steady state is achieved after 4 - 5 half-lives.

> A patient on digoxin therapy has a plasma digoxin concentration of 3.0 µg/L (3.9 nmol/L) and a plasma creatinine concentration of 125 µmol/L. She weighs 60 kg. It is decided to halve the digoxin dose. How long will it take to reach a new steady state?
>
> Steady state is reached after 4-5 half-lives. For digoxin, $t_{1/2}$ is normally about 40 hours, so it would take about a week to attain a new steady state. However, this time may be considerably lengthened in renal impairment. Despite the modest elevation in plasma creatinine, calculation of estimated creatinine clearance using the Siersback-Nielsen nomogram (Appendix Fig 3) gives a result of approximately 40 mL/min, suggesting that the half-life and time to reach steady state are likely to be twice the normal times. It would therefore be prudent to wait at least two weeks for a new steady state to be achieved before checking the plasma concentration again.

Example 6

Time for drug elimination

The half-life can be used to calculate how long it will take for a drug to be eliminated from the body after cessation of therapy – the concentration falls by 50% after one half-life, 75% after two half-lives, etc.

As part of treatment for an osteosarcoma, a 25 year old man received a high dose infusion of methotrexate at a rate of 14 g over six hours. Fluid and bicarbonate were given to maintain good urine flow and urinary pH above 8.0.

Plasma methotrexate concentrations measured at 8 and 24 hours following infusion were 112 and 7.0 μmol/L respectively. What is the half-life during the first 24 hours and what action should be taken?

The elimination rate constant is calculated from the two known concentrations and the time interval between them, and is in turn used to calculate the half-life (Eqs. 4.16 and 4.18)

$$k_d \quad = \quad \ln (C_1/C_2)/(t_1 - t_2) \qquad \text{(Eq. 4.16)}$$

$$= \quad \ln (112/7)/(24\text{-}8)$$

$$= \quad 2.773/16$$

$$= \quad \textbf{0.173} \ \ \textbf{h}^{\textbf{-1}}$$

$$t_{1/2} \quad = \quad \frac{0.693}{k_d} \qquad \text{(Eq. 4.18)}$$

$$= \quad \textbf{4 hours}$$

The patient has two pharmacokinetic risk factors after high dose methotrexate i.e. an initial $t_{1/2}$ of more than 3.5 hours and a 24 hour methotrexate concentration of more than 5 μmol/L. Folinic acid rescue therapy is necessary, and plasma concentrations should be monitored at least daily until less than 0.01 μmol/L.

Assuming a terminal half-life of 12 hours, estimate how much longer will it take for the methotrexate concentration to fall below 0.01 μmol/L?

For the concentration to fall from 7.0 μmol/L at 24 hours to 0.01 μmol/L requires a 700-fold fall i.e. between 9 and 10 half-lives (2^9 = 512, 2^{10} = 1024). A further 108-120 hours will therefore be required. A more precise estimate could be obtained by converting the terminal half-life of 12 hours back to a rate constant using Eq. 4.17 (0.058 h^{-1}) and then applying Eq. 4.15, giving a result of 113 h.

Case study 2

Optimal dosage interval

When a drug is given at regular intervals, the plasma concentration obviously rises and falls across the dosage interval, with the peak concentrations occurring soon after the dose has been taken and the trough concentrations immediately before the next dose. For most drugs, optimal effect is obtained with a relatively stable drug concentration across the dosage interval (aminoglycoside antibiotics are an exception to this general rule – see chapter 3) and it is therefore desirable to minimize fluctuations in concentration as far as practicable with convenient dosage regimes. This can be achieved if the dosage interval is less than or equal to the half-life of the drug. In this situation, changes in plasma concentrations are less than 50% of the peak concentration, and oscillate around the average steady state concentration. Oral administration of drugs leads to lower peak and higher trough concentrations than intravenous administration, and peak concentrations occur slightly later in the dosage interval.

When the dosage interval is much shorter than the half-life, as for example when amiodarone is administered daily, there will be little fluctuation of concentrations about the steady state concentration, which is primarily determined by drug elimination or clearance.

In contrast, when the half-life is much shorter than the dosage interval, for instance when using once-daily dosing for aminoglycoside antibiotics in patients with normal renal function, virtually all of the drug is removed from the body between each dose and peak concentrations correlate closely with the volume of distribution.

Prediction of plasma concentration after a loading dose or bolus of drug is given

The concentration at time 0 (C_0) may be obtained by rearranging Eq. 4.3:

$$C_0 \quad = \quad \frac{S \times F \times Dose}{V_d} \qquad \text{Eq. 4.19}$$

Since

$$C_t \quad = \quad C_0 \times e^{-k_e l t} \qquad \text{(Eq. 4.12)}$$

it follows that

$$C_t \quad = \quad \frac{S \times F \times Dose \times e^{-k_e l t}}{V_d} \qquad \text{Eq. 4.20}$$

A patient weighing 100 kg is given a 0.5 mg oral loading dose of digoxin. Assuming a normal volume of distribution of 7.3 L/kg and a clearance for digoxin of 146 L/24h, calculate the expected plasma concentration 12h later. (Salt conversion factor for digoxin = 1.0. Bioavailability of digoxin tablets = 0.62)

$$K_d \quad = \quad \frac{Cl}{V_d} \qquad\qquad\qquad \text{(Eq. 4.17)}$$

$$= \quad \frac{146/24}{7.3 \times 100}$$

$$= \quad 0.0083 \text{ h}^{-1}$$

$$C_{12} \quad = \quad \frac{1.0 \times 0.62 \times 500 \times e^{-0.0083 \times 12}}{7.3 \times 100} \qquad \text{(Eq. 4.20)}$$

$$= \quad 0.42 \times 0.905$$

$$= \quad 0.38 \text{ µg/L} \qquad (0.49 \text{ nmol/L})$$

Example 7

Prediction of plasma concentration at any time during a constant drug infusion

From equation 4.14, the steady state plasma concentration C_{ss} is given by:

$$C_{ss} \quad = \quad \frac{S \times F \times (Dose/\tau)}{Cl} \qquad\qquad \text{(Eq. 4.14)}$$

and the fraction of steady state achieved at time t after commencement of the infusion is $(1 - e^{-k_{el}t})$. Hence, the concentration at time t (C_t) is:

$$C_t \quad = \quad \frac{S \times F \times (Dose/\tau) \times (1 - e^{-k_{el}t})}{Cl} \qquad \text{Eq. 4.21}$$

As t increases, C_t will tend towards C_{ss}.

Prediction of plasma concentration following completion of an infusion

a. If the concentration has reached steady state, i.e., at least four half-lives, concentration at time t after stopping the infusion is given by:

$$C_t \quad = \quad C_{ss} \times \text{fraction remaining at time t}$$

$$= \quad C_{ss} \times e^{-k_{el}t}$$

Applying Eq. 4.14,

$$= \quad \frac{S \times F \times (Dose/\tau) \times e^{-k_{el}t}}{Cl} \qquad \text{Eq. 4.22}$$

b. If the concentration has not reached steady state, the concentration at time t_2 after stopping an infusion which has been running for time t_1

$$C_t \quad = C_{ss} \times (1 - e^{-k_{el}t_1}) \times e^{-k_{el}t_2}$$

$$= \frac{S \times F \times (Dose/\tau)}{Cl} \times (1 - e^{-k_{el}t_1}) \times e^{-k_{el}t_2} \quad \text{Eq. 4.23}$$

Prediction of steady state maximum and minimum concentrations

Trough samples (samples taken immediately before the next dose is given) give the most reproducible concentration measurements across a series of dosage intervals, as they are least affected by errors in timing or factors which may delay or accelerate drug absorption. They are, therefore, often the sample of choice for TDM in patients on chronic therapy. Trough samples are often used to give an estimate of steady state concentration, but if the variation across the dosage interval is of interest (for example if specific minimum concentrations for efficacy or maximum concentrations to avoid toxicity need to be maintained), it is possible to estimate the minimum and maximum concentrations between doses.

Maximum steady state plasma concentration (peak concentration)

$$C_{ssmax} = \frac{(S \times F \times Dose)}{V_d} \times \frac{1}{(1 - e^{-k_{el}\tau})} \qquad \text{Eq. 4.24}$$

This expression is a reasonable approximation only if the drug is rapidly absorbed and distributed – i.e. if the absorption and distribution times are short compared to the dosage interval.

Minimum steady state plasma concentration (trough concentration)

$$C_{ssmin} = C_{ssmax} \times e^{-k_{el}\tau} \qquad \text{Eq. 4.25}$$

where $e^{-k_{el}\tau}$ represents the decrease in concentration across the dosage interval τ.

Measured plasma concentrations can usually be substituted into the above equations to calculate V_d and k_{el} but this is not applicable to drugs for which the absorption and distribution rates are long in relation to the usual dosing interval. In this case the minimum concentration is similar to the steady state concentration and Eq. 4.14 can be used to determine clearance, since this is the major determinant of drug concentration under these circumstances.

Non-linear kinetics

Most of the drugs normally measured as part of a TDM service exhibit first-order kinetics, and their pharmacokinetic behaviour can be described using the equations described above. However, a few drugs, most notably phenytoin, do not conform to first order (linear) kinetics but instead show non-linear or zero-order behaviour, or a mixture of kinetic behaviours. In this situation, metabolic capacity is limited and the rate of elimination does not remain proportional to plasma concentration but falls off at higher drug concentrations due to saturation of the enzyme systems involved.

Since the problem is essentially one of enzyme kinetics and the capacity of enzyme systems, it follows that the mathematical model used is derived from the Michaelis-Menten equation, which dates back to 1913 and states that the rate (V) at which a substrate (concentration = S) can be metabolised by an enzyme is described by:

$$V = \frac{V_{max} \times S}{(K_m + S)}$$

where V_{max} is the maximum rate and K_m is the Michaelis-Menten constant (which can be shown to be equivalent to the substrate concentration at which V will be 50% of V_{max}). Substituting the average C_{ss} for substrate concentration and administration rate for V (since at steady state, rate of administration = rate of elimination):

$$\text{Rate of administration} = \frac{V_{max} \times C_{ss}}{(K_m + C_{ss})}$$

The rate of administration is also given by $(S \times F \times [Dose/\tau])$ (Eq.2). Hence:

$$S \times F \times (Dose/\tau) = \frac{V_{max} \times C_{ss}}{(K_m + C_{ss})}$$

and

$$C_{ss} = \frac{K_m \times S \times F \times (Dose/\tau)}{V_{max} - (S \times F \times (Dose/\tau))} \qquad \text{Eq. 4.26}$$

$$Dose = \frac{V_{max} \times C_{ss} \times \tau}{(K_m + C_{ss}) \times S \times F} \qquad \text{Eq. 4.27}$$

$$V_{max} = \frac{(S \times F \times (Dose/\tau)) \times (K_m + C_{ss})}{C_{ss}} \qquad \text{Eq. 4.28}$$

An epileptic patient is still having fits after taking 200 mg phenytoin sodium daily for two months. A blood sample, taken 12h post dose, showed a concentration of 7.5 mg/L (30 µmol/L). Assuming a K_m of 4 mg/L what dose is required to give a plasma level of 15 mg/L (60 µmol/L)?
Bioavailability = 1.0, Salt conversion factor = 0.92, Dose interval, τ = 24h

From Eq. 4.28, $\qquad V_{max} = \dfrac{(0.92 \times 1.0 \times 200/24) \times (4 + 7.5)}{7.5}$

$$= 11.76 \text{ mg phenytoin/h}$$

From Eq. 4.27, Dose for new $C_{ss} = \dfrac{11.76 \times 15 \times 24}{(4 + 15) \times 0.92 \times 1.0}$

$$= 242 \text{ mg}$$

(i.e. give 250 mg phenytoin sodium per day)

Note that as metabolism becomes saturated, a relatively small increase in phenytoin dose can lead to a marked increase in plasma concentration with consequent risk of toxicity. For example, if the patient in the above example were given another 50 mg per day (i.e. 300 mg/day in total), the predicted concentration would be 177 mg/L (700 mmol/L)! It is unwise to increase phenytoin dose by increments of more than 50 mg/day if the plasma concentration is > 5 mg/L (20 µmol/L) or by more than 25 mg/day if the plasma concentration is > 15 mg/L (60 µmol/L).

Example 8

Dosage prediction in practice

Dosage prediction can be approached in two main ways. The dosage regime to achieve a desired drug concentration can be estimated from average population pharmacokinetic parameters for bioavailability, salt fraction, clearance and volume of distribution obtained from the literature and supplemented by clinical data. Alternatively, measurement of one or more drug concentrations at appropriate times in the specific individual being studied allows calculation of patient-specific pharmacokinetic parameters using the equations above, which then allows further dosage optimisation using these parameters – TDM-assisted dosage optimisation.

Dosage prediction without drug measurement

In this situation average population estimates for the salt conversion factor, bioavailability, volume of distribution, clearance, elimination rate constant or half-life must be obtained from the literature. Accurate data are not always easy to find, and population estimates for these parameters often cover very broad ranges. If a drug is available in different formulations, data relating to the specific formulation must be used. These literature values are then supplemented with clinical data relating to the individual, such as age, sex, weight, body surface area, renal, hepatic or cardiac function, smoking and/or alcohol history and other medications which may alter clearance. Correction of literature pharmacokinetic values for these factors is not always straightforward, but this approach can give an initial estimate of the dose required to achieve a given concentration, which can subsequently be refined using the following method.

Dosage prediction with drug measurement

Drug concentrations obtained at known times in relation to dosing are invaluable in improving the accuracy of dosage prediction based on population parameters. It is vital to ensure that the starting data is accurate, for example that the time the drug was actually taken is known (rather than the time when it was supposed to be taken). Drug concentration values for the individual patient can then be used in the equations above to derive patient-specific pharmacokinetic parameters and allow more accurate predictions of the plasma drug concentrations that would be obtained on different dose regimes.

Nomograms for dosage prediction

Nomograms may be useful for calculating some of the parameters used in dosage prediction such as body surface area, creatinine clearance or theophylline clearance. They may also be used in place of pharmacokinetic equations, for example in optimising phenytoin or gentamicin regimes.

Nomograms for calculating body surface area (BSA)

These are modelled on the formula of DuBois and DuBois:

BSA (in m^2) = $Wt^{0.425}$ x $Ht^{0.725}$ x 0.007184

where weight (Wt) is in kilograms and height (Ht) in centimetres. They are available for children and adults. An alternative approach to calculating body surface area is to use the formula derived by Mosteller in 1987:

BSA (m^2)   = $\sqrt{(Ht \times Wt / 3600)}$

(Ht in centimeters and Wt in kilograms as before).

Nomograms for estimating creatinine clearance
Various nomograms are available, although only those which consider age, sex and body weight give sufficient accuracy of prediction. The Siersback-Nielsen nomogram, introduced in 1971 is commonly used, and is reproduced in an amended form in Figure 3 of the Appendix.

Nomograms for estimating clearance of theophylline
It is reasonably easy to predict the clearance (and hence dosage regimes) for drugs whose elimination is largely determined by renal function and can therefore be characterised by creatinine clearance. For other drugs, where metabolism is a major component of the elimination pathway, clearance may be affected by a wide range of genetic, environmental, physiological and pathological factors, and dosage prediction is therefore more complex. Theophylline is a good example of such a drug. Approximately 90% of absorbed theophylline is metabolised by hepatic microsomal enzymes and clearance is therefore highly variable. Jusko et al investigated a large number of possible factors and produced a nomogram to predict theophylline clearance including subdivisions on the basis of age, sex, obesity, smoking and alcohol habits, presence of congestive heart failure, and use of oral contraceptives, benzodiazepines, barbiturates or marijuana. The original nomogram is therefore highly complex, but it may be simplified somewhat, as shown in Figure 4.3 and has been incorporated into various computer-based dosage optimisation systems. A series of clearance multiplication factors, first described by Powell *et al* in 1978 and augmented by Chrystyn in 1984, are shown in Figure 4.4 and may be more practical for routine use.

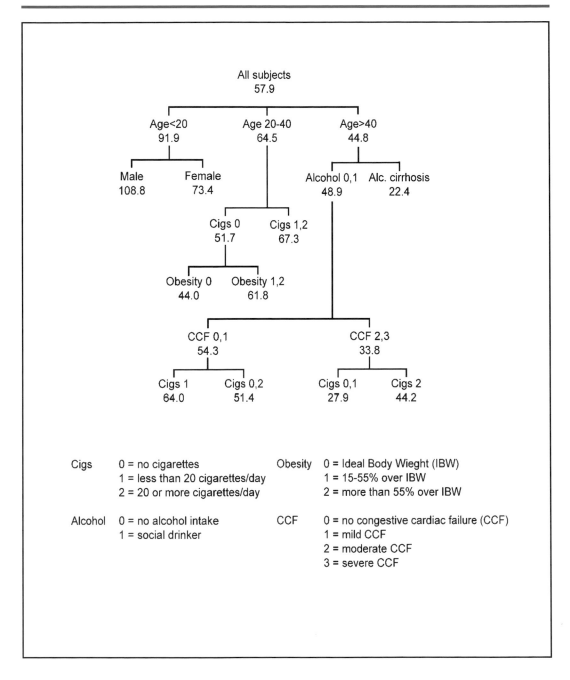

Figure 4.3 Abbreviated version of the Jusko theophylline clearance nomogram with clearance values in mL/h/kg ideal body weight

Clearance multiplication factors for use in estimating theophylline	
Contributing conditions	**Clearance multiplying factor**
Smoking (> 20 cigarettes per day)	1.6
Congestive heart failure (CHF)	0.8
Severe CHF	0.4
Acute pulmonary oedema	0.5
Hepatic cirrhosis	0.5
Chronic obstructive airways disease	0.8
Chronic alcohol intake	0.5
Male < 18 years old	1.8
Female < 18 years old	1.2
Concurrent barbiturates	1.3
Concurrent erythromycin	0.5
Concurrent cimetidine	0.6
Concurrent benzodiazepines	1.3
Concurrent tricyclic antidepressants	1.2
The theophylline clearance is multiplied by the appropriate factor	

Figure 4.4 Clearance multiplication factors for use in estimating theophylline

Nomograms for optimising phenytoin therapy at steady state

As previously discussed, the metabolic pathway for phenytoin can be saturated at therapeutic concentrations, producing a non-linear relationship between dose administered and the resulting plasma concentrations. As the point of saturation nears, small dosage increments may be required to optimise treatment without inducing toxicity, and a number of nomograms are available which allow dosage prediction based on one, or usually two, steady state phenytoin concentrations.

A simple nomogram using a single steady state plasma concentration to predict the dose required to achieve a desired phenytoin concentration was published by Richens in 1975 and subsequently refined by Rambeck et al in 1979. The refined nomogram, shown in Figure 4.5, was constructed from a study of patients aged between six and seventy-two. K_m was found to be independent of age and the nomogram can therefore be used for all age groups. However, it does not allow assessment of an individual patient's values for K_m or V_{max} and may under- or over-estimate dose requirements in many cases, since K_m can vary widely between patients.

Rambeck nomogram for phenytoin optimisation

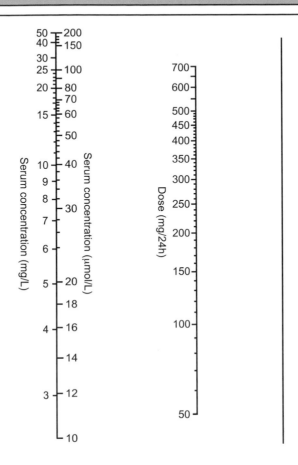

Given a single reliable serum concentration on a given daily dose of phenytoin sodium, the dose required to achieve a desired level can be predicted. A line is drawn connecting the observed concentration (left-hand scale) with the dose administered (centre scale) and extended to intersect the right-hand vertical line. From this point of intersection another line is drawn back to the desired serum concentration (left-hand scale). The phenytoin dose required to produce this concentration can be read off the centre scale.

Remember that this nomogram will give misleading predictions if the serum concentration measurement is inaccurate, if the patient is not fully compliant, or if concurrent treatment has been changed since the level has been taken.

As in the use of all phenytoin nomograms, accurate measurement and exemplary patient compliance are essential to yield accurate predictions. Further, between drug measurement and dosage adjustment there should be no changes in drug binding to plasma proteins or in concurrent medication.

More accurate individual predictions may be obtained using two dose levels and associated plasma concentration measurements. Such data allow estimation of K_m and V_{max} from either the Ludden (1977) or Mullen (1978) plots, the former requiring some prior calculation of drug clearance. The direct linear plot of Mullen also permits graphical interpolation of the dose required to achieve a desired phenytoin concentration; details for its use are given in Figure 4.6.

Direct linear plot of Mullen for phenytoin optimisation

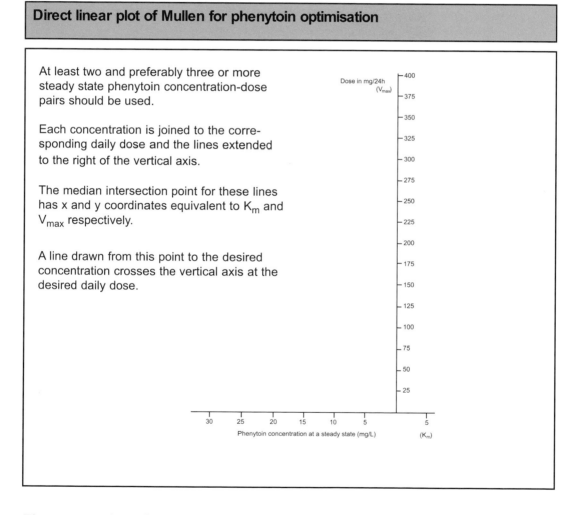

At least two and preferably three or more steady state phenytoin concentration-dose pairs should be used.

Each concentration is joined to the corresponding daily dose and the lines extended to the right of the vertical axis.

The median intersection point for these lines has x and y coordinates equivalent to K_m and V_{max} respectively.

A line drawn from this point to the desired concentration crosses the vertical axis at the desired daily dose.

Dose in mg/24h (V_{max})

Phenytoin concentration at a steady state (mg/L)   (K_m)

Figure 4.6 Direct linear plot of Mullen for phenytoin optimisation

Figure 4.5 Rambeck nomogram for phenytoin optimisation

A more sophisticated approach is exemplified by the orbital plot of Vozeh *et al* (1981), as shown in Figure 4.7. This can be used in situations where either one or two data pairs are available and is based on a Bayesian adjustment procedure, described in more detail below. When only one data set is available, the probability contours, which are superimposed on the basic direct linear plot, allow estimation of the most probable individual K_m and V_{max} values. The highest probability contour through which the line passes gives an indication of how unusual an individual patient's kinetics are. Lines that do not cross the central ellipse therefore represent unusual kinetics and should be treated with suspicion. When the line is very steep, indicating a low concentration despite a high dose, compliance is questionable whereas a flat line, indicating a relatively high phenytoin level for a low dose, may suggest overcompliance, hepatic disease or a drug interaction.

Vozeh orbital plot for phenytoin optimisation

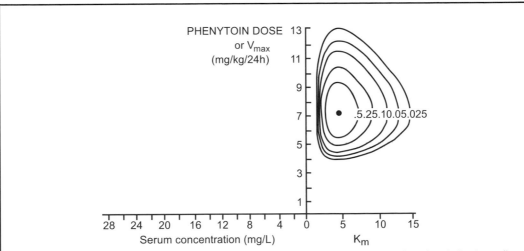

1. If one steady state phenytoin concentration is available draw a line joining the daily dose (in mg/kg/24h phenytoin sodium) to the measured concentration (in mg/L).
2. Find the innermost ellipse which is dissected by the extrapolation of this line.
3. The midpoint of the line crossing this ellipse is an estimate of the most likely K_m and V_{max} combination for this patient.
4. Drawing a line from this midpoint to the desired plasma concentration allows the appropriate phenytoin dose to be read off the y axis.
5. When two or more Cp_{ss}-dosage pairs are available the nomogram can be used like that of Mullen to determine patient-specific values of K_m and V_{max}, obtained from the parameter values at the intersection(s) of lines drawn for each pair.

Figure 4.7 Vozeh orbital plot for phenytoin optimisation

A 25 year old man had been treated for grand mal epilepsy for five years following brain damage sustained during a motor cycle accident. Initially his seizures had been well controlled on a dose of 150 mg phenytoin sodium bd, however one month ago he had four fits. The trough phenytoin concentration was 10 mg/L (40 μmol/L). He weighed 70 kg and had normal renal and liver function.

Assuming good compliance, use the Rambeck nomogram (Figure 4.5) and Vozeh orbital plot (Figure 4.7) to estimate an appropriate dose to achieve a phenytoin concentration of 15 mg/L (60 μmol/L).

The Rambeck nomogram gives a recommended dose of 350 mg phenytoin sodium per day. The orbital plot recommends a dose of 340 mg per day. Four weeks later a second sample is received, with a request form stating "recent ataxia and nystagmus on 200 mg bd phenytoin. ? toxic."

Using the estimates of K_m and V_{max} from the orbital plot calculate the steady state concentration for this regime.

From Fig 4.7, K_m = 5.0 mg/L (20 μmol/L) and V_{max} = 455 mg/24h.

Applying Eq. 26,

$$C_{ss} = \frac{K_m \times S \times F \times (Dose/\tau)}{V_{max} - (S \times F \times (Dose/\tau))}$$

(assume F = 1, and S may also be taken as 1, as doses of phenytoin sodium were used in the Vozeh plot)

$$C_{ss} = \frac{5.0 \times (400/1)}{455 - (5.0 \times (400/1))}$$

using 24h (1 day) as the unit of time.

$$= \frac{2000}{455 - 400}$$

$$= 36.4 \text{ mg/L} \quad (145 \text{ μmol/L})$$

Case study 3

Nomograms for gentamicin administration

The use of nomograms for prediction of gentamicin dosage has been radically altered by new developments in the way gentamicin is used. Older nomograms have been rendered largely obsolete by the change to once-daily (or less frequent) dosage regimes, based on the work of Nicolau *et al.* (the 'Hartford' nomogram) (Figure 4.8). The measured plasma concentration after an initial standard dose (7 mg/kg) is used to predict the subsequent dosage interval, rather than varying the dose itself. The original version of the nomogram simplifies the actual decay curves into straight lines for ease of use. It should be noted that the nomogram is not applicable in children, and in pregnancy or patients with ascites, endocarditis, cystic fibrosis, burns, neutropenia, or with creatinine clearance < 20 mL/min. The approach is illustrative, and computer programs based on less aggressive dose regimes (e.g. 5 mg/kg) and on more accurate modelling of the decay curve are also available.

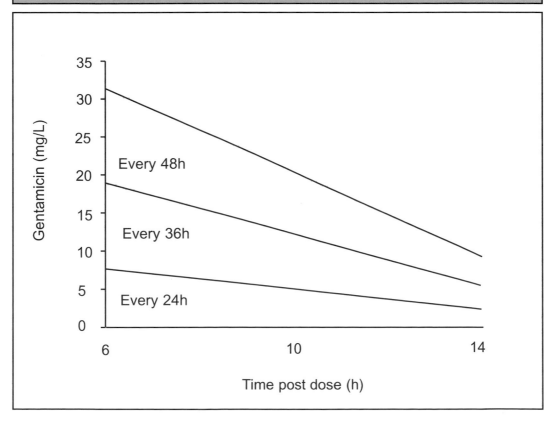

Hartford nomogram for prediction of gentamicin dosage

Figure 4.8 Hartford nomogram for predicting gentamicin dosage

Computer-assisted dosage prediction

Software to assist dosage prediction ranges from automated forms of simple pharmacokinetic equations to more complicated systems which employ population pharmacokinetics, Bayesian statistical theory, maximum likelihood estimation and neural networks.

Population pharmacokinetics

Population pharmacokinetics describes inter-individual pharmacokinetic variability in terms of a number of components called fixed and random effects. The fixed effects are the average population values of pharmacokinetic parameters which may, in turn, be a function of patient characteristics such as age, sex, height and weight, underlying pathology such as renal or hepatic impairment and other influences on drug metabolism such as concomitant drug therapy, smoking and alcohol consumption. The random effects are those which remain after all fixed effects are accounted for, including inter-subject variability within the population, intrasubject variability, analytical error and other sources of error. The population pharmacokinetics approach has formed the basis of a number of the nomograms which have been described in the preceding sections.

A different technique treats the population rather than the individual as the unit of analysis. By studying more people but fewer data points per person, a more representative sample of the target population can be obtained. Kinetic and demographic data can be analysed simultaneously by software such as NONMEM (Nonlinear Mixed Effects Model) which evaluates the observed concentration and time data in terms of the fixed and random variables described above. Collection of such information has been undertaken for a variety of drugs and can lead to increased efficiency of dosage adjustment, often based on a subsequent Bayesian feedback procedure.

Bayesian principles in pharmacokinetics

As previously indicated, the equations used in this chapter may be used to estimate drug doses in the absence of measured drug concentrations, using population pharmacokinetic parameters from the literature adjusted for patient characteristics such as gender, weight, age and serum creatinine concentration, or they may be used to estimate individual patient pharmacokinetic parameters from measured concentration data. Both these methods have disadvantages when used in isolation, and a combination of the two approaches is often preferable.

The Bayesian approach to dosage prediction combines the *a priori* (population pharmacokinetics) approach with measured concentration data to produce a refined (*a posteriori*) estimate of population parameters, taking into consideration the variability of the population parameters and the variability of the serum concentration measurement. The Bayesian approach mimics human thought in that, before we take a course of action, our intuition tries to foresee all the possibilities which might arise. We then judge how likely each one is, based on what we see and on our past experience.

Bayes' theorem was developed by the Rev Thomas Bayes (1702-1761) and published posthumously in 1763. It may be stated as:

Posterior probability = Prior probability x likelihood ratio

where literature values for population pharmacokinetics give us the prior probability and we use measured concentration data to provide a likelihood ratio estimation and give us the posterior probability (best estimate of the individual's pharmacokinetic parameters).

As more analytical data are obtained, less statistical weight is given to initial population estimates (the prior distribution) and more to the most recent information (the posterior distribution). This produces a more precise model to estimate the dose necessary to achieve a desired plasma concentration profile.

This approach forms the basis of many neural network systems or other computer programs for dosage optimisation. Such systems have been described and made commercially available for a variety of drugs and are valuable in experienced hands, particularly when complicated drug regimes have been used. Care should however be taken in their use, particularly by people who do not understand their underlying principles and limitations. The output from dosage prediction programs is only as good as the data fed into them, and dose predictions should always be checked by an experienced practitioner before being used clinically.

Further reading

Camps-Valls G, Porta-Oltra B, Soria-Olivas E, Martin-Guerrero JD, Serrano-Lopez AJ, Perez-Ruixo JJ, *et al.* Prediction of cyclosporine dosage in patients after kidney transplantation using neural networks. IEEE Trans Biomed Eng 2003; **50:** 442-8.

Chrystyn H, Mulley BA, Peake MD. Precise individualisation of theophylline dosage using a nomogram and Bayesian analysis and dependence of accuracy on preparation used.In: Turner-Warwick M, Levy J, eds. New perspectives in theophylline therapy. London: Royal Society of Medicine International Congress and Symposium Series 1984; **78:** 117-127.

Cockcroft DW, Gault MH. Prediction of creatinine clearance from serum creatinine. Nephron 1976; **15:** 31-41.

Dubois D, Dubois EF. A formula to estimate the approximate surface area if height and weight be known. Arch Int Med 1916; **17:** 863-871.

Jusko WJ, Gardner MJ, Mangione A, Schentag JJ, Koup JR, Vance JW. Factors affecting theophylline clearances: age, tobacco, marijuana, cirrhosis, congestive heart failure, obesity, oral contraceptives, benzodiazepines, barbiturates and ethanol. J Pharm Sci 1979; **68:** 1358-1366.

Levey AS, Bosch JP, Lewis JB, Greene T, Rogers N, Roth D. A more accurate method to estimate glomerular filtration rate from serum creatinine: a new prediction equation. Ann Intern Med 1999; **130:** 461-70.

Ludden TM, Allen JP, Valutsky WA, Vicuna AV, Nappi JM, Hoffman SF *et al.* Individualization of phenytoin dosage regimens. Clin Pharmacol Ther 1977; **21:** 287-293.

Mosteller RD. Simplified calculation of body surface area. N Engl J Med 1987; **317:** 1098.

Mullen PW. Optimal phenytoin therapy: a new technique for individualizing dosage. Clin Pharmacol Ther 1978; **23:** 229-232.

Nicolau DP, Freeman CD, Belliveau PP, Nightingale CH, Ross JW, Quintiliani R. Experience with a once-daily aminoglycoside program administered to 2,184 adult patients. Antimicrob Agents Chemo 1995; **29:** 650-655.

Rambeck B, Boenigk HE, Dunlop A, Mullen PW, Wadsworth J, Richens A. Predicting phenytoin dose - a revised nomogram. Ther Drug Monit 1979; **1:** 325-333.

Rowland M, Tozer T. Clinical Pharmacokinetics, Concepts and Applications. Philadelphia: Lea and Febiger, 3rd edn, 1995: 24-5.

Schwartz GJ, Haycock GB, Edelmann CM, Spitzer A. A simple estimate of glomerular filtration rate in children derived from body length and plasma creatinine. Pediatrics 1976; **58:** 259-263.

Siersbaek-Nielsen K, Hansen JM, Kampmann J, Kristensen M. Rapid evaluation of creatinine clearance. Lancet 1971; **1:** 1133-1134.

Thomson AH, Whiting B. Bayesian parameter estimation and population pharmacokinetics. Clin Pharmacokinet,1992; **22:** 447-467.

Whiting B, Kelman AW, Grevel J. Population pharmacokinetics. Theory and clinical applications. Clin Pharmacokinet 1986; **11:** 387-401.

Vozeh S, Muir KT, Sheiner LB, Follath F. Predicting individual phenytoin dosage. J Pharmacokinet Biopharm 1981; **9:** 131-146.

Yamamura S. Clinical application of artificial neural network (ANN) modeling to predict pharmacokinetic parameters of severely ill patients. Adv Drug Deliv Rev 2003; **55:** 1233-51.

Chapter 5

Optimising drug therapy for individual patients

Chapter 1 has illustrated the potential for between-individual variation in drug metabolism, and has emphasised the need for measures of drug efficacy and drug toxicity. The measurement of drug concentrations in biological fluids (classical TDM) plays a considerable role in this process, but is not the only weapon in the armoury of markers of drug action. The drive towards personalized medicine (selection and administration of drugs specifically tailored to the individual patient) requires the application of TDM in conjunction with measures that can predict response before a drug is given and those that are able to detect differences in the clinical response to a particular drug concentration (pharmacodynamic differences). These measures are currently less well developed than classical TDM, but are poised to play an important role in individualizing drug therapy in the future. The purpose of this chapter is to outline the basis, scope and future potential of approaches not based on measurement of drug concentrations – specifically, pharmacogenomics and pharmacodynamic biomarkers.

TDM is essentially based on population data – 'target ranges' that produce a satisfactory clinical effect in the majority of patients studied. It is good at describing and compensating for inter-individual variation in the pharmacokinetic processes described in Chapter 1, and for many drugs (where pharmacokinetic variation dominates), TDM is essential in achieving therapeutic efficacy and avoiding toxicity. Many applications of this process are described in detail in Chapter 2. However, as already mentioned, TDM has its limitations. It is not very suitable for drugs with a high pharmacodynamic variability – where the clinical response to drug action does not correlate well with the plasma concentration, due to drug interactions at the receptor level, variable receptor density or affinity, or the effects of illness and poor perfusion or penetration of drug to the site of action. TDM is also limited if active metabolites are present which are not measured by the assay system used, but are responsible for part of the clinical effect. Finally, TDM by its very nature can provide no information on an individual's susceptibility to a drug before the drug has been given, nor can it provide useful information about the likelihood of adverse drug reactions in a particular individual.

Awareness of these limitations, and powerful developments in human genetics and our understanding of the mechanisms of drug action, have stimulated research in two new fields – the use of genetic information to predict drug metabolism and response (*pharmacogenomics*) and the development of biomarkers to provide an objective measure of an individual's clinical response to therapeutic intervention. The combined use of all three techniques (pharmacogenomics, biomarkers and drug concentration monitoring) is likely to be the key to personalized medicine, but offers considerable scientific, informatics and educational challenges.

Pharmacogenomics

Classical TDM uses concentration measurements of drugs in body fluids to guide optimization of therapy and minimise adverse consequences, but this approach relies inherently on a recognition that something is wrong with the initial drug or dose and that action needs to be taken to correct or improve the situation. Pharmacogenomics holds out the potential to get it right the first time – identifying the right drug and the right dose for the individual patient without the need for the cycle of trial dose/assess response/revise dose/re-assess response that has so often characterised the therapeutic process.

The term *pharmacogenetics* has been used since the 1950s to describe the study of inherited differences in drug metabolism and response, and is strictly used to discuss the influence of a single gene or phenotype. More recently, in the context of the Human Genome Project, the term pharmacogenomics has been coined to refer to the general study of genes determining drug behaviour, and thus has a wider field of reference. The two terms do, however, tend to be used interchangeably.

The essence of pharmacogenomics is linking differences in gene structure (polymorphisms) to differences in drug metabolism and response, i.e. connecting genotype with phenotype. Polymorphisms of the enzymes of drug metabolism may have a range of effects, including altering the proportion of drug which is inactivated on the first pass through the liver after absorption (effectively altering the amount of drug delivered to the systemic circulation), changing the elimination characteristics of a drug (prolonging the half-life or changing the proportion of active metabolites), and altering the drug concentration-effect relationship. Study of these effects and their consequences has many potential applications, including improved drug development, individualisation of therapy, reduction of adverse drug reactions and defining susceptibility to medication or the potential for addiction – all of which have the potential to reduce iatrogenic disease and make a considerable impact on the cost of health care.

Adverse drug reactions (ADRs) were stated in a 1998 study to be the fourth most common cause of death in the USA and a Bandolier article in 2002 estimated the cost of ADRs to the UK National Health Service to be 4% of available bed-days and approximately £380 million per year. Many of the drugs most frequently cited in ADR reports are metabolised by one or more enzymes with variant alleles known to cause altered metabolism, which implies considerable scope for reduction in ADRs by intelligent use of genetic information. The increasing availability of susceptibility testing will drive this process rapidly, since a patient who learns that they have suffered an ADR, which could have been avoided if the physician had performed a simple test before prescribing the drug, will have a strong case for legal action. The prescribing information for atomoxetine, a drug used in attention deficit-hyperactivity disorder in children, now states that poor metabolisers of the drug will have much higher blood concentrations, which may lead to adverse reactions, and that laboratory tests are available to identify susceptible individuals. As this information enters the public domain, the demand for testing for genetic variants in drug metabolism is expected to rise dramatically.

The clinical applications of pharmacogenetics are extensive. A comprehensive exposition is beyond the scope of this chapter and recent reviews should be consulted. Some examples of applications are in anticoagulation (polymorphism of the cytochrome P450 (CYP) 2C9 isoform), oncology (thiopurine methyltransferase polymorphisms and the serum Her2/neu receptor), psychiatry (polymorphisms of the CYP 2D6 isoform), epilepsy, pain control and other areas.

Thiopurine Methyltransferase

Thiopurine methyltransferase is a paradigm for the use of genetic information in this way. Thiopurine drugs (azathioprine, 6-mercaptopurine and thioguanine) have an established role as immunosuppressive agents in a range of clinical conditions. Adverse effects of the drugs lead to withdrawal of therapy in up to a quarter of patients, and life-threatening myelosuppression may occur. Thiopurine methyl transferase (TPMT) catalyses the methylation of 6-mercaptopurine and its precursors to inactive mercaptopurines (Figure 5.1) and competes with the primary metabolic pathway which leads to pharmacologically active product (6-thioguanine nucleotides, 6-TGN). Individuals with high TPMT activity produce less 6-TGN and are at risk of therapeutic failure, while individuals who are deficient in TPMT activity produce more of the cytotoxic drug and are susceptible to toxicity. Approximately 1 in 10 of the population are heterozygous for TPMT deficiency, and 1 in 300 are completely deficient. Prior knowledge of TPMT status avoids exposure of these individuals to potentially fatal treatment, and identification of hypermethylators reduces the incidence of therapeutic failure. Screening for TPMT status appears to be cost-effective and it would now be difficult to defend a case of fatal azathioprine-induced marrow suppression in a TPMT-deficient individual who had not been screened prior to starting treatment.

Mercaptopurine metabolism

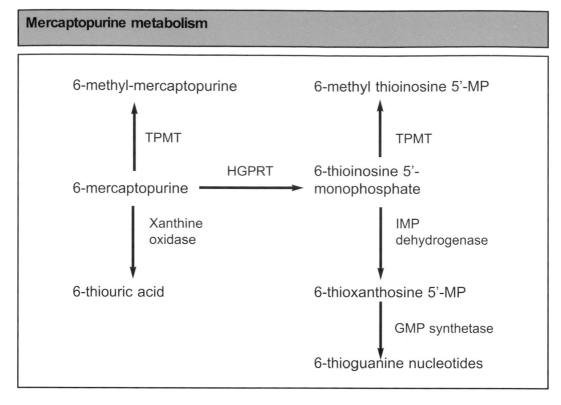

Figure 5.1 Mercaptopurine metabolism

Homozygous deficiency of the enzyme is associated with specific mutations, most commonly G460-A (Ala 154 - Thr) and A719-G (Tyr 240 - Cys) which lead to the TPMT*3 genotype at chromosome 6p 22.3. Both phenotyping (measurement of enzyme activity) and genotyping have been used to enable safe and effective therapy. Since genotyping cannot detect hypermethylators and runs the risk of missing individuals with TPMT deficiency caused by unknown or double-mutant alleles, phenotyping is preferred for clinical purposes, although genotyping has an important confirmatory role.

Cytochrome P450 (CYP450) polymorphisms

The cytochrome P450 mixed-function oxidase system is responsible for Phase 1 oxidation of a range of xenobiotics prior to Phase 2 conjugation reactions. Cytochrome P450 is a family of haem-related proteins found in smooth endo-plasmic reticulum, chiefly in the liver and the gut. There are more than 30 different forms in humans, which are characterised by sequence similarities. The individual enzymes are named in families and subfamilies, so in the case of the CYP450 2D6*4 allele, CYP450 represents the cytochrome P450 superfamily, the figure 2 the family and the letter D the subfamily, and the figure 6 denotes the individual isoenzyme. The figure 4 after the star identifies the specific allele.

In the area of drug metabolism, different cytochrome P450 isoenzymes have different, albeit often overlapping, specificities for groups of drugs (Figure 5.2). Thus determining the phenotype or genotype for a particular isoform may give information about the individual's ability to handle a range of drugs metabolised by that isoform, increasing the power of pharmacogenetic information. The CYP2D6 isoform is the most extensively characterised polymorphic drug-metabolizing enzyme, with more than 75 allelic variants described. More than 15 of these variants encode an inactive enzyme or no enzyme at all, and other variants encode enzyme with reduced, normal or increased enzyme activity, leading to patients who are poor, normal or extensive metabolisers of the substrate drugs. CYP2D6 is involved in the metabolism of approximately 30% of all approved drugs.

CYP isoforms in drug metabolism	
CYP1A2	tricyclic antidepressants antipsychotics selective serotonin release inhibitors sedatives
CYP2C9	anti-epileptics anticoagulants
CYP2D6	debrisoquine tricyclic antidepressants antipsychotics selective serotonin reuptake inhibitors anti-arrhythmics anti-hypertensives morphine derivatives
CYP2C19	barbiturates tricyclic antidepressants sedatives
CYP3A4	tricyclic antidepressants antipsychotics selective serotonin release inhibitors sedatives

Figure 5.2 Example specificities of CYP isoforms in drug metabolism

A commercially available microarray (Amplichip CYP450, Roche Diagnostics) now permits profiling of 33 alleles of the CYP2D6 and 3 alleles of the CYP2C19 genes in a single assay.

Warfarin and related anticoagulants are metabolized by the CYP2C9 isoform of cytochrome P450. The gene for CYP2C9 contains 9 exons coding for 490 amino acids, and each variant isoform is a result of a single nucleotide polymorphism leading to a single amino acid substitution (Figure 5.3). The *2 allele is found in 6% of Caucasians and 6% of Asians, and produces 5-fold lower warfarin clearance. The *3 allele is found in 8% of Caucasians, and produces 25-fold lower warfarin clearance. Pre-dose genotyping of the CYP2C9 gene can therefore inform prescribing and avoid excessive anticoagulation in susceptible patients.

CYP2C9 polymorphism

Isoform	Amino acid at position		
	144	359	360
CYP2C9*1	Arg	Ile	Asp
CYP2C9*2	Cys	Ile	Asp
CYP2C9*3	Arg	Leu	Asp
CYP2C9*4	Arg	Thr	Asp
CYP2C9*5	Arg	Ile	Glu

Figure 5.3 CYP2C9 polymorphism

Translation of the promise of pharmacogenomics into clinical practice will require more than just the evidence base to support usage of the genetic tests and more general availability of those tests. There will need to be much greater understanding by prescribing physicians of the basis of the tests and the meaning of the results. There are ethical issues to consider, and the Nuffield Council on Bioethics has produced a useful summary. However, the ethical issues are considerably more manageable and easier to address than those in other areas of genomics, such as screening for disease susceptibility. Clinical biochemists have the knowledge and skills necessary to support routine pharmacogenetic testing, and will have a vital role in developing protocols and provision of testing. The US National

Academy of Clinical Biochemistry (www.nacb.org) is producing a Laboratory Medicine Practice Guideline consensus document (expected 2008), addressing the practical issues of bringing pharmacogenetic testing into the routine laboratory.

Biomarkers

Pharmacogenetics undoubtedly has a huge role to play in tailoring drug therapy to the individual patient, as indicated above. However, as stated in the Introduction to this chapter, not all the factors affecting drug metabolism are genetic. Pharmacogenetics can predict the genetic influences on metabolism, classical TDM can give information about the concentration of active substances in relevant body fluids and define individual pharmacokinetics, but there is still a role for biomarkers of the actual effect of a drug to define the individual's pharmacodynamic response. A biomarker may be broadly defined (US National Academy of Sciences) as 'a xenobiotically-induced variation in cellular or biochemical components or processes, structures or functions that is measurable in a biological system'. An alternative definition, provided by the NIH/FDA Biomarkers Definition Working Group is 'a characteristic that is objectively measured and evaluated as an indicator of normal biological processes, pathogenic processes or pharmacological response(s) to a therapeutic intervention'.

These definitions are necessarily very broad, and within their overall scope, could cover anatomical or histological properties, genes, proteins, metabolites, mRNA, imaging properties, cell counts etc. For the purposes of this discussion, a narrower definition of TDM biomarkers has been proposed by Clarke and McMillan: 'a biochemical measurement that can be used to determine efficacy, extent of toxicity, or individual pharmacodynamics for a therapeutic agent'.

The obvious application is where the desired clinical application is in itself a change in a biochemical parameter, e.g. cholesterol for lipid-lowering drugs or glucose for hypoglycaemic agents. To extend the application of biomarkers to other conditions, it is necessary to identify a biological analyte that correlates with the pharmacodynamic effects of the drug, effectively becoming a surrogate for some clinical outcome. Hitherto, most such markers have been markers of toxicity rather than of therapeutic efficacy (e.g. urinary N-acetylglucosamine as an index of tubular damage caused by drugs with a nephrotoxic action or liver enzymes as indicators of hepatotoxicity), but there has been increasing interest in biomarkers which give direct information about the efficacy of a drug. Red cell 6-thioguanine nucleotides (see section on thiopurine methyltransferase above) are an effective biomarker of thiopurine drug effect, and a number of biomarkers have been described in the field of transplantation immunology to measure the effect of immunosuppressive agents (see page 107).

Ciclosporin (CsA) acts by inhibition of calcineurin activity preventing the transcription of several cytokine genes which are necessary for T-cell activation, and there is a close temporal relationship between CsA concentration and calcineurin inhibition when calcineurin activity is analysed in peripheral blood leucocytes or in whole blood. Calcineurin activity is thus an effective surrogate biomarker of immunosuppressant activity.

Similarly, the action of the immunosuppressive drug mycophenolate mofetil is based on reversible inhibition of inosine 5′-monophosphate dehydrogenase (IMPDH) by mycophenolic acid (MPA), and quantitative measurement of IMPDH activity in whole blood generally correlates well with plasma MPA concentration and can provide additional information over drug concentration measurement in some cases.

An immune cell function assay, the Cylex Immunoknow™ assay, is now commercially available for the measurement of global immune response in transplant patients receiving immunosuppressive therapy. The assay detects cell-mediated immune responses in whole blood after a 15-minute incubation with phytohaemagglutin as stimulant. ATP produced by stimulated cells is measured luminometrically and characterises the level of cellular immune function.

Integrating information

Pharmacogenetics and new biomarkers provide exciting adjuncts to conventional drug concentration monitoring in creating truly individual therapeutic regimes. Integrating the information available from all three strands is a complex challenge, and will undoubtedly require decision support software and effective strategies for presenting the information in an accessible format to those responsible for patient care. Pre-treatment pharmacogenetic profiling will allow identification of individuals who are likely to be particularly susceptible or resistant to a proposed treatment strategy, allowing better choice of starting dose or the use of a different drug. However, the effect of factors like disease, age and other drugs means that pharmacogenetics can never tell the whole story, and a combination of biomarkers of effect and monitoring of drug or metabolite concentrations will be needed to complete the picture and enable truly personalized medicine.

Further reading

Biomarkers Definitions Working Group. Biomarkers and surrogate endpoints: preferred definitions and conceptual framework. Clin Pharmacol Ther 2001; **69:** 89-95.

Clark W, McMillin G. Application of TDM, pharmacogenomics and biomarkers for neurological disease pharmacotherapy: focus on antiepileptic drugs. Personalized Medicine 2006; **3:** 139-149.

Eichelbaum M, Ingelman-Sundberg M, Evans WE. Pharmacogenomics and individualized drug therapy. Ann Rev Med 2006; **57:** 119-37

Nuffield Council on Bioethics. Pharmacogenomics: Ethical issues. London: Nuffield Council on Bioethics, 2003.

Oellerich M, Marten MJ, Armstrong VW. Biomarkers: The link between therapeutic drug monitoring and pharmacodynamics. Ther Drug Monit 2006; **28:** 35-38.

Sanderson J, Ansari S, Marinaki T, Duley J. Thiopurine methyltransferase – should it be measured before commencing thiopurine drug therapy? Ann Clin Biochem 2004; **41:** 294-302.

Shastry BS. Pharmacogenomics and the concept of individualized medicine. Pharmacogenomics J 2006; **6:** 16-21.

Appendix

Nomogram for calculating body surface area in children

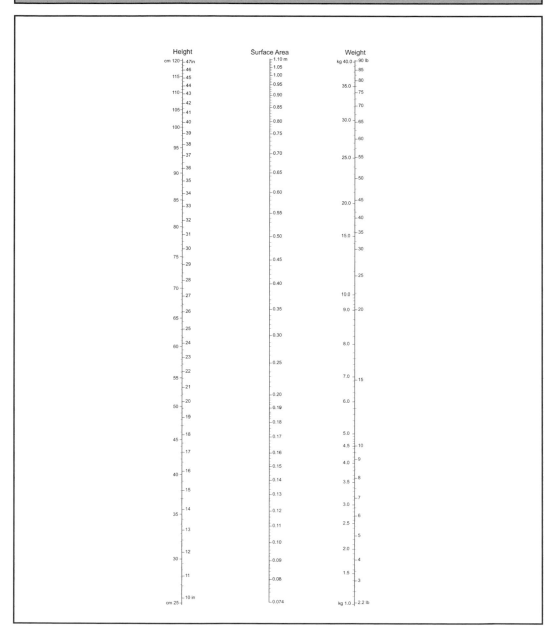

Figure 1 Nomogram for calculating body surface area in children (from Dubois et al, Arch Int Med 1916; 17: 863-871 with permission).

Nomogram for calculating body surface area in adults

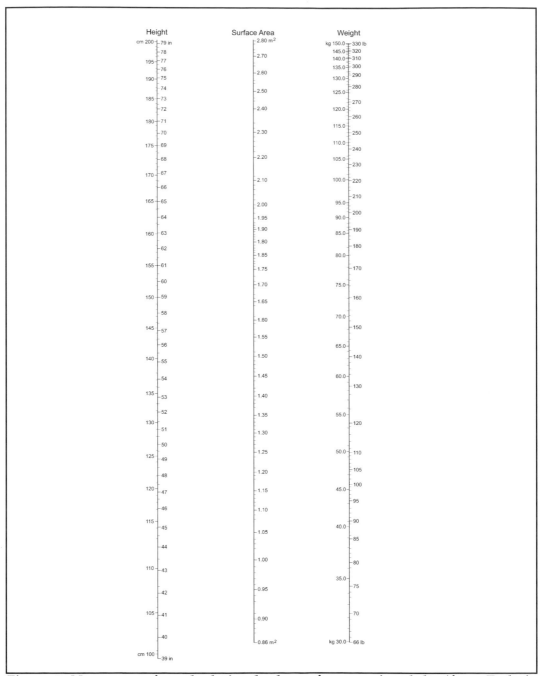

Figure 2 Nomogram for calculating body surface area in adults (from Dubois et al, Arch Int Med 1916; 17: 863-871 with permission).

Nomogram for calculating creatinine clearance

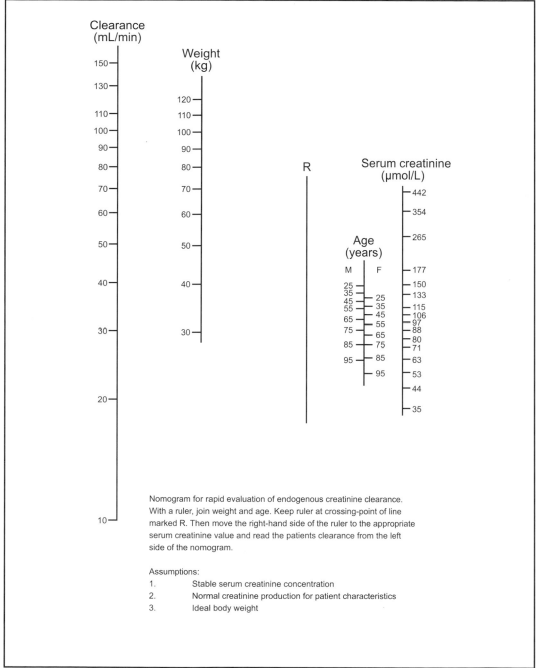

Clearance (mL/min)

150 —
130 —
110 —
100 —
90 —
80 —
70 —
60 —
50 —
40 —
30 —
20 —
10 —

Weight (kg)

120 —
110 —
100 —
90 —
80 —
70 —
60 —
50 —
40 —
30 —

R

Age (years)

M   F

25 —
35 —   25 —
45 —   35 —
55 —   45 —
            55 —
65 —
            65 —
75 —
            75 —
85 —

95 —   85 —

            95 —

Serum creatinine (µmol/L)

442
354
265
177
150
133
115
106
97
88
80
71
63
53
44
35

Nomogram for rapid evaluation of endogenous creatinine clearance. With a ruler, join weight and age. Keep ruler at crossing-point of line marked R. Then move the right-hand side of the ruler to the appropriate serum creatinine value and read the patients clearance from the left side of the nomogram.

Assumptions:
1.   Stable serum creatinine concentration
2.   Normal creatinine production for patient characteristics
3.   Ideal body weight

Figure 3 Nomogram for calculating creatinine clearance (from Siersbaek-Nielsen K *et al*, Lancet 1971; 1: 133-134 with permission).

Glossary of terms
(with abbreviations)

Adherance	The extent to which a patient takes medication as prescribed.
Apparent volume of distribution	see Volume of distribution.
Area under the curve (AOC)	Area beneath the plasma concentration time plot. A measure of the amount of drug absorbed.
Bioavailability (F)	The fraction of administered dose which reaches the systemic circulation.
Chirality	The potential of a molecule to exist in two (or more) different stereoisomeric forms.
Clearance (Cl)	The ability of the organs of elimination to remove drug from the body. Defined as the theoretical volume of drug which can be completely cleared of drug in unit time.
Compliance	see Adherance
Dosage interval	The period of time between individual doses.
Elimination half-life	see Half-life.
Elimination rate constant (k_d)	Fraction of the total amount of drug in the body which is cleared in unit time.
Excipient	Inert material in a tablet or capsule.
Extraction ratio	Fraction of drug removed from blood or plasma as it passes through an organ (hence hepatic extraction ratio, etc).

First-order kinetics	Process by which the amount of drug in the body diminishes logarithmically over time. Rate of elimination is proportional to the plasma concentration.
First-pass metabolism	Removal of drug from the plasma after absorption and before reaching the systemic circulation usually in the liver.
Free fraction (a)	Fraction of drug not bound to protein in plasma.
Half-life	Time required for the plasma concentration to fall to half its original value. The alpha or initial half-life is the half-life representing distribution of drug into the tissues. The beta or elimination half life is the half life representing elimination of drug.
Loading dose (LD)	Initial dose given to achieve a given plasma concentration rapidly.
Maintenance dose	Dose given to replace drug lost from the body and maintain a steady plasma concentration.
One compartment model	Common model of drug behaviour which assumes that drug distributes equally to all parts of the body.
Pharmacodynamics	Study of the biochemical and physiological effects of drugs, and their mechanisms of action.
Pharmacokinetics	Study of the absorption, distribution, metabolism and excretion of a drug and its metabolites in the body.
Plateau	Stable concentration of drug in plasma found at steady state.

Salt conversion factor (S) (salt fraction)	Fraction of active drug present in a particular salt or compound.
Steady state	Point at which the rate of administration of drug is balanced by the rate of elimination.
Target range	The plasma concentration range over which a drug exhibits therapeutic benefit with minimal toxicity in the majority of patients.
Therapeutic index, or therapeutic ratio	The margin between the concentration at which a drug exerts a therapeutic effect and the concentration at which toxic effects are observed.
Therapeutic range	see Target range.
Two compartment model	Model of drug behaviour involving initial, rapid distribution to one volume of distribution (for example, the plasma space), followed by slower distribution to another volume (for example, tissue fluids).
Volume of distribution (V_d)	The volume of a compartment necessary to account for the total amount of drug in the body if it were present throughout the compartment at the same concentration found in the plasma.

Index